Dr. Quinn's

BLUEPRINT

Unlock Your True Potential

DR. TIMOTHY QUINN

On Fridays, I pick up my daughter from school. Today was special, because I had the exciting news about starting the book. I reminded her of all our previous conversations about what the book represented. We talked about my desire to help my fellow Mississippians achieve better health by knowing the importance of being proactive in regards to their health. We also talked of the strategy that would be illustrated throughout the book—to not only inform of the problem but to provide an applicable solution. My daughter told me that this book would also help people outside the borders of Mississippi. She looked me in the eyes and said, "Dad, this book will help the world! I believe in you, Dad."

CONTENTS

PREFACE

My motivation to write this book resulted from my observation of phenomenal life-changing improvements people experienced after acquiring the basic concepts illustrated in this presentation. I have practiced family medicine in my home state, Mississippi, for the last ten years. Prior to practicing as a family physician, I had the opportunity to experience many life lessons that taught me the concepts that I have shared directly with patients and the general public during public speaking engagements, television and radio interviews, and print publications in various papers and magazines. There have been many other presentation opportunities in social media. I strongly believe that everyone has a purpose, and getting the opportunity to fulfill it is the greatest fulfillment of ones' life. Over the years, my purpose has evolved from increasing health awareness to increasing self-awareness. I have been delightfully enlightened to learn that when you are self-aware, your overall actions will change to give you better health, better finances, better relationships, and an overall better life for you and your loved ones.

The constant theme of the concepts discussed in this book involves self-awareness, and understanding that we can positively impact many life scenarios. In many instances, we unfortunately accept conditions that are less than optimal. We don't take steps to improve the unfavorable situations, because we don't believe that we can do anything to achieve improvement. With the explanations illustrated via factual accounts of my life and the lives of people I have observed, the reader will better understand the "I can" thought process. The first step of becoming fully aware of the situation and all the factors involved is most important. Once you understand your position and the consequences of not acting—or acting in a way that will not improve the situation—you can act effectively to change the situation for the better! My advice is to try not to get too excited as you discover how to reach your true potential, and live the life that you have always deserved.

Many of my childhood memories are as clear today as when they happened. Many of these memorable events change our lives by influencing our way of thinking, and play a large part in the development of who we are. A person's thought process has the largest controlled impact on their life. We cannot control our genetics or the financial status of our parents, but we can control how we react to life's challenges. If someone has a strong genetic predisposition to a specific medical condition, this cannot be controlled. This same individual can, however, control how they react to this potential problem. An example would be a person with a strong family history of diabetes, with complications to include a parent that may have gone blind or lost a limb due to this condition being poorly controlled. This same individual may choose to aggressively adhere to a healthy diet and exercise program. This person may develop diabetes despite his positive lifestyle, but have it controlled with oral medications with no complications. This person may not have to take insulin, and develop complications due to a poor lifestyle with bad food choices and a lack of exercise. The same scenario can occur with a person with a strong family history of cancer avoiding terminal cancer by choosing to get timely cancer screenings. This could theoretically include a lady whose mother died of breast cancer that was diagnosed late. This lady could potentially get a mammogram, and receive a diagnosis and treatment if the mammogram is positive before the cancer can spread, avoiding a premature death. We can choose to act in every aspect of our lives to impact the outcome of most situations for the better.

When I reflect on my childhood, and memorable occurrences that helped me develop an empowered belief in my ability to change unfavorable situations, I feel encouraged. For many people, a lack of action to make situations better is not due to a lack of desire, but a lack of understanding and belief. I believe that everyone has a purpose, and as a primary care physician practicing for over twelve years in Mississippi, I have been blessed to understand my purpose. Some people ask why I work for so many hours, and I always truthfully respond that I have been fortunate to get up every morning, and have the privilege of helping others. With a smile I inform them, "I haven't worked a job since college." I must admit that the hours can be taxing at times, but the reward of helping someone understand that they can make a difference is the greatest compensation I could imagine. This empowering thought process that I share with patients daily include life challenges and many scenarios in addition to medical problems. Examples include helping married couples understand that they cannot control their spouse, but they can control themselves. This includes a wife with a husband who may not behave the way she desires. With a "can do" attitude, the wife is led to understand that she has a better chance of a successful marriage by actively changing her approach from an angry spouse to a loving one. With this new approach, she now uplifts her husband as opposed to tearing him down. In many scenarios, the husband will react positively. There are scenarios where the spouse is a lost cause, but the person must actively choose to make every possible attempt to save the marriage as opposed to feeling helpless. We cannot ultimately control situations but by acting, we make our chances better.

1

THE BEGINNING

"WHERE OTHERS SAW JUST ANOTHER POOR, DUMB KID FROM SMALL TOWN MISSISSIPPI, **MY COMMANDER SAW UNTAPPED POTENTIAL** BURIED BENEATH YEARS OF **CRITICISM, BAD HABITS, AND MISDIRECTION."**

BLUEPRINT: THE BEGINNING

Growing up in the small, impoverished, rural community of McComb, Mississippi, I had no mentors or aspirations other than graduating high school. There were no plans or dreams after graduation during that period in my life. The reality of most men of our community would include finding a low-paying job, father children with a small chance of marriage, and hang out on the weekends. My family was poor with limited resources. Living in a single-parent home, we relied on government assistance and the focus was on survival. There was little attention given to living beyond McComb. It wasn't that my mother didn't want the best for my brother and me; she was simply limited in her view of what was possible. That viewpoint coupled with poverty and low self-esteem created a recipe for me to become another statistic.

I give many seminars to students to encourage them to strive for excellence. I tell them my story as motivational encouragement to demonstrate that they can have a better future. On many occasions, I am asked how I was able to get on a better path. I then tell them of the pivotal time in my life when I decided to attend college. My initial reason for attending college was to have, what I perceived to be, fun. This perception resulted from a visit to Alcorn State University during my junior year of high school. At the urging of my cousin, who was a freshman at this university, I went to Alcorn for a weekend to participate in college life. We attended many parties, a football game, and had more fun than I had ever imagined. It was something different, and though my motives were wrong, something awakened inside of me to see myself "outside" McComb.

I remember returning to McComb that Sunday night. I walked into my home and announced to my mom, "Your baby boy is going to college!" With great excitement, great excitement, my mom signed me up for the College Admission Test (ACT). Because of my lack of preparation, I performed poorly on the test. Due to my low grade-point average, and my low College Admission Test score, I was allowed admission on academic probation.

After being advised by my uncle to join the military reserve to pay for college, since it was too expensive for my family to afford, I enlisted in the Army National Guard. I performed well in the eight-week basic training course in South Carolina due to my athletic history of playing football and running track. However, I ran into problems during my Advanced Individual Training course in San Antonio, Texas. My commander in Texas saw something in me. Where others saw another "poor dumb kid from small town Mississippi," my commander saw untapped potential that was buried underneath years of criticism, bad habits, and misdirection.

Because I had scored above average on the enlistment altitude test, I was placed in the medical field to serve in the military. Still, my academic performance in San Antonio was horrible. Because of my continued poor academic performance, despite my physical successes, I was faced with being deployed to the Middle East since the country was currently at war and my unit back in Mississippi was facing deployment. My commander informed me that he was recommending me to be transferred to Fort Benning, Georgia to do an expedited infantry course to allow me to serve in the Desert Storm War on the front line as an infantry soldier. As he talked, I was only hearing, "Tim, you are going to die!" It was in that moment that my life changed. I saw that if I didn't take control of my life, my outcome would be death. Many people at various points in their lives are faced with a similar scenario—do or die!

In total desperation, I pleaded with my commander to allow me to start over with the incoming class. He agreed to give me one more chance, and with that chance he held me accountable. When we are forced to deliver, we begin to reevaluate what's important in life. To me, it was life itself. Even then, I didn't quite have the right motives, but it was another "spark" that awakened my pursuit of living beyond limits.

I studied around the clock and did not hang out as I had earlier, prior to this meeting with destiny. To my surprise, I scored a high score on every exam. The war soon ended, and I was allowed to start college the following fall semester. I entered college on academic probation status, but due to my new understanding of my ability and potential, I graduated with honors and was eventually accepted into medical school.

How did all this happen? I worked hard, saw success, and repeated it time and time again. By going off to the military and college, I had the opportunity to be exposed to people from all over the world with dreams that I would have never imagined. By now, while applying myself academically, I had a firsthand confirmation that I could perform just as well as any of my new acquaintances. Through this process, I developed the audacity to believe in myself.

Like many of my fellow Mississippians, I have had many family members suffer from not being proactive in their medical care. This was the strongest motivating factor for me in becoming "The People's Doctor."

My grandfather died of metastatic prostate cancer, meaning that the cancer had spread to multiple areas in his body from the original source. If he would have been diagnosed and treated early, he would have had a good chance of being saved. I loved my grandfather and respected him. He was a great man and a leader in his community, serving as the pastor of three churches. He believed in prayer, and allowing God to do His will. Yet, he wasn't a huge advocate of going to doctors or hospitals. When he started to develop symptoms, he did not follow up with medical care as advised. My grandmother would call me in California, where I was doing my residency, and tell that my grandfather was sick. She would ask me to encourage him to go to the doctor, and tell me scenarios of him fainting and having blood in his urine. Still, he wouldn't comply.

During his last days in the hospital, my grandfather told me that God visited him and told him that he was wrong on how he viewed doctors and medical care. At that moment, my grandfather understood that God uses people, even today, to perform miracles on earth.

Though my grandfather didn't mentor me, or push me to dream beyond McComb as a child, he forever changed the course of my life in this one conversation. Many times, we are looking for something but we already possess it. For my grandfather, it was I. And for me, it was he. We both, though from two different generations, held the "keys" to each other's next level of thinking. It was on his deathbed that he unlocked the door to my purpose that longed to be free. He told me that God told him that I was to be a tool, a soldier, and a miracle in His army. My grandfather further explained that I was a planned weapon in God's arsenal that was to be used to do His will, not mine. And that is a lesson all dreamers must not forget.

My humble beginnings and sincere desire to see people live long, healthy lives never would make me a "traditional" doctor. And I now understand that is ok, because greatness doesn't have a set code or specified definition. He reminded me that I was always different and misunderstood. He reminded me that I did not look or act like the other kids, which resulted in the playground beatdowns early on. But he explained how he watched me adapt over the years and become a leader of my peers, a leader of children of few luxuries living in one of the poorest towns in our country.

My grandfather helped me realize that everything I have gone through, as a child and a young adult, had not been wasted. It prepared me to go into the poorest neighborhoods as a doctor and feel comfortable communicating with people. My level of comfort helped the people feel comfortable with me, resulting in them freely expressing their concerns, which allowed me to provide good medical care. Since returning to Mississippi to start a medical practice, after my residency in Los Angeles, I have provided medical care to a great number of people from all walks of life. Many who, like my grandfather, lacked the appreciation and trust of medicine and doctors. I have been blessed to work toward removing the "fear" of going to the doctor, and replacing it with an "I look forward to going to the doctor" attitude.

CHAPTER

2

CHOOSING TO ACT

"I REMINDED HER THAT THE ENTIRE PREMISE OF THE BOOK WAS TO IDENTIFY A PROBLEM, IDENTIFY THE STEPS NEEDED TO CORRECT THE PROBLEM, DEVELOP A PLAN TO SOLVE THE PROBLEM, AND EXECUTE THE PLAN TO ELIMINATE THE PROBLEM."

BLUEPRINT: MENTAL FITNESS & CHOOSING TO ACT

While meeting with my publicist to discuss the progress of the book, I received a text from a good friend who had been proofing some of the information that I had been sending to my publicist in preparation for the book. I called her while driving home. She was very upset because she had gained five pounds while trying to lose weight by eating healthier. My first response was a question. I asked her if she could help me summarize what my book was going to be about. After a short discussion, we both agreed that the book was about taking steps to improve situations we feel are less than optimal. I praised her for the attempt to eat healthier, and she credited me for motivating her by sharing my ideas. I reminded her that we previously talked about the fact that achieving her ideal weight would be more likely by incorporating a healthier lifestyle with a better diet and an increase in her activity level. She admitted that she had not taken any steps to improve her lack of exercise. I reminded her that the entire premise of the book included identifying a problem, then identifying the steps toward the solution, and lastly, execution of the plan. She told me that she had identified that she wants to reach a healthier weight, and giggled as she admitted that a big part of her motivation was to improve her appearance. She further admitted that she had identified steps of eating healthier and increasing her activity in the form of exercise as a way to reach her desired weight. I asked her to put the phone down, change into tennis shoes and comfortable clothing, and report to the nearest walking trail. I explained to her that talking about it only wasted time and did not make the situation better. I asked her to text me a picture of her shoes on the trail in no less than forty-five minutes. Forty-five minutes later, I got a picture of tennis shoes on what appeared to be a tar surface. Assuming this was the walking trail, I got a warm feeling in my heart for my friend.

I often ask my patients what stopped them from executing the plan they had previously decided to acquire their desire. An example was a discussion I had with a pre-med undergraduate student. We had previously discussed how he could increase his chances on getting accepted to a medical school. I told him of how I had contacted the local medical school my sophomore year in college, and asked if I could get an appointment with the dean of admissions. I further told him of how I had showed up for the appointment early, wearing a suit I had purchased from the Salvation Army because I wanted to wear a nice suit but could not afford to purchase one from a department store. I told him how the dean had admitted that she was not clear why I was scheduled to meet with her. The student was impressed when I told him how I first thanked her for agreeing to meet me, and further explained that I wanted to know what I could do to increase my chances of getting accepted to her medical school. I told the student how I had researched and memorized many facts about the medical school and the dean of admissions prior to the meeting. The student listened as I told him how the dean was very flattered as I praised many of her accomplishments, and impressed that I knew so much about the medical school. I explained to the student how I told her of my experience prior to college as a medic with my deployed Army National Guard unit during the Desert Storm War. I told the student that I shared with the dean a true scenario I used on my medical school mission statement—my first experience of knowing that I was destined to become a doctor when I made a finger splint for a soldier out of two plastic spoons. I elaborated how the other soldiers praised me and started calling me Doc. I explained that this was the most fulfilling time in my life, because I was able to use my previous training to help another person. I told the student that this was a pivotal time in my life when I was blessed to know my purpose. A year later, I met with the student. He told me that he often thought of contacting the school since our meeting last year, but failed to make the call. He apologized, and admitted that this would definitely help his chances. I asked him to wait in my office as I went to the next room to make a call. I returned five minutes later with the new dean of admissions on the phone. Three weeks later, he met with the dean. One year later, he received his acceptance letter to the medical school.

Did the meeting with the dean help the student's chances of getting accepted to the medical school? Did walking on the day my friend complained about her weight gain eventually helped her get closer to her desired weight? I feel confident that you will agree that the actions did not hurt their chances. We do not have total control over any situations. I remember a recent scenario, which occurred during a routine run to achieve better health: I was caught in a thunderstorm and thought I could be struck by lightning, which would definitely not improve my health. I thought of how I could not control the fact that it started lightning or that a car could run off the curve and hit me. The friend that started her walking program after the motivational phone call could have twisted her ankle resulting in less mobility and increased weight. The dean could have been insulted, and misunderstood the student as being arrogant for having a doctor call him and arrange for a meeting. Even though we are not in full control, we have to do whatever we can to make our chances better. In situations involving poor outcomes due to uncontrollable factors, we have to continue to act to achieve our desires.

I once needed a job while in college when my car broke down. After applying to a grocery store across the street from my apartment, and being told that there were no jobs available, I showed up and started bagging groceries. When the manager asked what I was doing, I told him I wanted to volunteer until a job became available. I was told I was either a "crazy person" or the future employee of the month. I was hired on the spot. I took a risk, knowing that I could have been embarrassed if the security had escorted me out of the store.

In many scenarios, it can be risky to act toward achieving your desires. It is risky to take out student loans to go back to school. It is risky to tell your feelings to the person you desire to be with. It is risky to walk into a gym full of fit people and start exercising. It is risky to tell your friends that you don't want to join them for the buffet. It is risky to show up early for work and out-perform others on your job. It is risky to sit in the front of your class, answer all the questions, and turn your work in early. Many of us fear being laughed at. We fear that our peers will say that we are "kissing tail." We take comfort in blending in, and not take the risk of being noticed by acting differently. If you research some of the most successful people, their personal history will reveal that many people misunderstood them initially. These leaders were called many names like nerds, misfits, outsiders, crazies, etc.

Early on, I decided that I was not going to allow other people's opinions to determine my destiny. Once you realize that many people are going to discourage your efforts due to their own insecurities, you will have conquered an obstacle that many cannot. Take that step that you know will help you reach your goals.

CHAPTER

3

PERSISTENCE

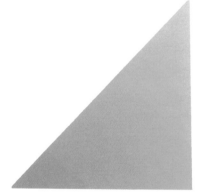

I HELD HER HANDS,
LOOKED HER STRAIGHT IN HER EYES,
AND SAID AS FORCEFULLY AS I COULD
**"WINNING COMES FROM PERSISTENCE
& COMMITMENT".**

BLUEPRINT: MENTAL FITNESS & PERSISTENCE

Miss Jones asked me how she could be healthier. She was recently diagnosed with diabetes. She was prescribed an oral medication, and was told she did not need the insulin. I did, however, inform her that she might need the insulin later if she did not lose weight with a better diet and consistent exercise. Miss Jones told me that she had many unsuccessful attempts of losing weight in the past; she could not stick to it. She told me that she always gave up, and told herself that she would be successful one day. She then started to tell me how she used to work out and eat healthy. I immediately asked her to stop. I told Miss Jones that "used to" is a loser's term. I informed her that she had to develop a winner's mentality. I made it a point to stress that winners do not always win, but they never quit. I looked her in the eyes, took her hands, and told her that winning is a result of persistence and commitment.

I told Miss Jones about my daughter who wanted to be a cheerleader. She tried out for the cheerleader's squad, but learned that the other girls trying out were getting private cheer lessons from coaching and tumbling staff for the last six months. She asked me to sign her up for the lesson, which I quickly learned did not come cheap. I was in the process of purchasing a new car, but decided to delay it for two months and use the money for the private cheer lessons. She would receive the lessons three days a week for two months, leading to the tryouts. On the night of the tryouts, she received the notification that she did not make the team. I immediately told her that I had to go for a drive. She called me while I was driving to ask if she could continue the lessons. Totally confused, I asked her, "Why would you continue the lessons when you did not make the team?" Saffron told me that she wanted to continue the lessons because she was going to make it next year. I almost drove the car off the road, and it is good that I didn't because I still don't have a new car. But even though a great deal of my finances went toward the lessons, I now spend my Friday nights cheering for my cheerleader daughter. I explained to Miss Jones that this was a winner's mentality. To not give up is key.

I told Miss Jones that the next step was understanding why she needed to lose weight. I told her of a Christmas morning in my hometown of McComb, MS. It was very cold and my uncle was confused why I went for a run in the cold. He told me that I did not enjoy any of the good food, including the desserts. He told me that I was crazy. He went on to tell me that if he were a doctor, he would be as fat as he wanted and still have all the dates he wanted. I explained to him that my dedication to fitness had nothing to do with desires for dates. I then shared a story with him about a recent patient who desperately wanted to lose weight to attend her high school twenty-year reunion, and impress a classmate who never acknowledged her. She told me that he was recently divorced, and she now had her chance after twenty years. She was a twenty-six dress size and was able to get down to size sixteen over six months, during which she participated in a dedicated diet and exercise regimen. After the reunion, she returned to the office and sadly informed me that the guy did not even remember her, and did not show any interest in her. With tears in her eyes, she told me that she was a big fat loser. I explained to her that she was a winner. I told her this was because she set a goal to become healthier, and was successful. I explained that all her hard work and dedication was not in vain. I reminded her that initially she was on insulin and oral medications for diabetes, which was not controlled. I also reminded her that she was on three different blood pressure medications and a cholesterol medication. I then reminded her of how we were able to stop the insulin, and only take pills for the diabetes, which was now well controlled. I also reminded her that her blood pressure and cholesterol, for the first time, is now controlled. This control is accomplished with only one pill for blood pressure and one pill for cholesterol. I told her that she might be able to get off her medications if she maintains this persistent diet and exercise regimen. I told her that she did not get the big date with the superficial loser from her high school but she was a winner, because she set a goal, and stuck to it to receive the success of better health.

Achieving better health involves getting into the right mindset first. It also includes setting yourself up to win. Some of the examples I give to my patients involve lessons I learned from my own experiences. Some of these experiences involved me accomplishing other goals, but the same principle stood. Your environment has a great impact on the success of whatever goal you wish to accomplish. Your environment includes the people around you. When I started medical school, I initially hung out with my fraternity brothers from two neighboring colleges in Nashville and Fisk. Not surprisingly, my grades reflected my associations. The first request my dean gave was to decrease the time I spent with people not in medical school, and start spending more time with medical students. He told me that the other medical students would have a positive impact on my graduating. I noticed that hanging out with medical students did help me do better in school. Statements from my new peers such as, "Let's check out the new cadavers in the gross anatomy lab on Friday night" helped. This was different than the usual statement of, "Let's check out the Greek show after party this Friday night!" I advise the people who are trying to achieve a healthier lifestyle to surround themselves with people trying to accomplish the same objective. I told a patient that she did not want to meet up with friends after church who suggested going to the new buffet restaurant. I suggested she should find friends who suggested going to the new gym and having a smoothie.

CHAPTER

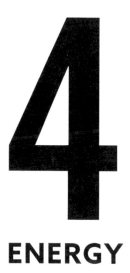

ENERGY

"**WHEN WE CHOOSE TO ENGAGE IN STRESSFUL SITUATIONS** THAT ARE AVOIDABLE, WE ARE CHOOSING TO **EXPOSE OUR PHYSICAL AND MENTAL SYSTEMS** TO UNNECESSARY ATTACKS."

BLUEPRINT: ENERGY

According to the first law of Thermodynamics, energy cannot be created or destroyed. Energy can change forms, and energy can flow from one place to another. I often think of this concept in relation to humans and fate. I have many patients who accept and maintain negative energy. This negative energy manifests in the enablers to cause many problems, mentally and physically. We all have the ability to choose. Recently, my yardman charged me for an outrageous amount for work he did on my yard without my approval. My assistant that reviewed the charge asked if I wanted her to give him a piece of her mind for this unrequested bill. After telling her this was unnecessary, she smiled, and asked if I wanted to deliver the message. I explained to her that this would cause unnecessary stress, and to simply search for a new yard keeper. When we choose to engage in stressful situations that are avoidable, we choose to expose our physical and mental systems to this unnecessary process. Biochemical hormones are released into our circulatory system that can cause increased blood pressure, fatigue, chest pain, anxiety, and for some, depression. There are other physical and mental symptoms experienced by different people depending on the person and the level of stress.

We cannot avoid all stressful situations, but we can choose to avoid the unnecessary ones. When we are faced with a situation that cannot be avoided, it is advised to systematically approach it as carefully as possible. This way of thinking further allows us to have a greater control of our lives. A technique that has really been helpful to me is to always try to focus on the solution as opposed to the problem in unavoidable, less-than-optimal situations. I remember once listening to a speaker talk about a salesman who had been sent to a country in Africa to sell running shoes. He contacted the company after arriving, and requested to be returned home because the people of this country, for the most part, only wore sandals. The speaker stated that he was an intern in the company and overheard the conversation. He stated that he asked to take the salesman in the African country's place. After having a record-breaking year in shoe sales, he explained that he credited his success to the fact that he saw a situation where no one had running shoes, and he saw the opportunity to help them understand how beneficial these shoes would be to assist them in their activities requiring fast mobility such as hunting.

We cannot control our genetics, but we can control how we choose to use our gifts inherited from our parents. I often use the basketball superstar Kobe Bryant to illustrate this concept when addressing audiences. I explain that his father was a great basketball player who played in the professional league. I further explain that he inherited height and agility from his parents. I point out that I did not inherit any of the physical traits that Kobe did. I then point out that Kobe choose to practice at a much higher level, and dedicate more time to perfecting his skill level according to persistent reports from his teammates. He took his genetically inherited skill, and chose to use his energy to perfect his performance. We all have this option.

When I was in medical school, there was a student we will call John Doe. Both his parents were specialists in medicine. My parents did not attend college. John Doe was from a long line of professionals with his parents being third-generation doctorate level professionals. Initially, John was the only medical student I would hang out with on the weekends. We would go to parties at the neighboring colleges and hang out with undergraduate students. Early on, I met with my academic advisor, and was informed that I had to improve my grades. John continued to hang out, but I had to decline the fun parties. At the conclusion of medical school, John was at the top of the class with the best grades. I passed, but was far from the top. John had the ability to look at a page in a book briefly, understand it, and answer any question about the content. He also had to the ability to retain this information for the examination, and continue to retain this information years later when taking board exams. I had to review, take notes, and restudy the information many times with hours of work. He had genetic traits for brilliance.

I chose to divert my energy from partying to studying. This was a conscious choice. When the dean told me that I might not pass, I did not choose to use my energy getting angry at the dean or the university. I remember a student who would come to the library every night and complain how everything was unfair. He would further talk about how everyone was against him, and wanted to have this conversation with other students who were trying to study. I once asked him if he would consider what would happen if he spent all the time he was complaining, studying. I suggested his choice of how he spent his time would result in better grades. I ran into him at a conference two years ago. He explained how his grades turned around after he stopped focusing on what was wrong. He eventually graduated, two years late, but he graduated when he chose to use his energy to study.

CHAPTER

5

CHRONIC ILLNESS

"WHEN MOST HEAR THE WORD CANCER, THEY IMMEDIATELY THINK DEATH SENTENCE."

BLUEPRINT: FIGHTING CHRONIC ILLNESS

J ust as you can positively impact your outcome regarding your weight, your career, your relationships, and many other scenarios of your life, you can also positively impact your outcome of a diagnosis of cancer. When we hear the word cancer, most people immediately think it is a death sentence. We hear that cancer has no cure. Many patients tell me that they do not want to have cancer. Many patients tell me that they do not want to get a colonoscopy, lab tests for prostate cancer, or a mammogram, because they don't want the diagnosis of cancer. Many of us feel that we are helpless and have no control. We can sometimes find comfort by not wanting to know. Hopefully, this information will help you feel empowered, and help you understand that you do have some control. Our Creator blessed us with the ability to choose, and the choosing to increase our information can help us make better choices.

I recently spoke to an audience, encouraging them to take control of their health. I told of a recurring scenario that involved me in a public place, such as a grocery store. The last incidence took place in a Wal-Mart store. A lady I had no memory of ever seeing before, approached me. She had tears in her eyes as she gave me a hug. Uncomfortably, I asked her to what do I owe this nice hug. She told me that I saved her life. She told me how she watched me do an interview on television about two ladies with two different outcomes of cancer. She reminded me of the first lady who saw me in the office with the complaint of back pain. This lady hadn't seen a doctor in over ten years, and it turned out that the back pain was cancer that had spread to her backbone and other organs in her body. The second lady was seen for a routine physical, and scheduled for a routine screening mammogram. The second lady's mammogram had microscopic calcifications or early stage cancer that was diagnosed before it had the opportunity to spread. This second lady had an outpatient procedure where the cancer was removed, and the pathological and radiological studies confirmed it. The first lady's situation could have been the same, but she neglected to get her timely screenings and was diagnosed too late. The lady in the grocery store told me that this interview motivated her to get the screening. Although she was diagnosed with cancer, it was diagnosed early. The lady in the Wal-Mart had the same scenario as the second patient that was diagnosed early, and was treated. She told me that the information saved her life.

Diagnosing cancer early, in many cases, can lead to successful treatment. I recently spoke of a popular windshield repairman in our local area who calls himself Dr. A. Whenever a rock or any object strikes your car windshield, you call Dr. A. He comes and patches it up. Dr. A informs that waiting or delaying his windshield-saving procedure can result in the loss of your windshield, because, as he explains, the crack grows with time. Once the crack has grown to a significant size, his routine repair no longer works. With some financial pain, we can get another windshield, but we cannot get another life. Diagnosing cancer with timely screenings drastically changes outcomes for many Americans every year. This holds true for breast cancer with screening mammograms, prostate cancer with blood PSA (prostate specific antigen) and DRE (digital rectal exam) tests, and colon cancer with screening colonoscopies.

This "catch it early" concept also holds true for many medical conditions, including heart disease. I have a presentation I provide to address this subject titled "the two trucks." I ask the listeners to imagine two eighteen wheelers that are required to travel six hours daily for years to make a delivery. I ask them to imagine that both trucks have an operation span of an average six years, give or take two years. This means some trucks will break down and become inoperable at four years and others will last for eight years. I emphasize that between four and eight years, most trucks become inoperable. I ask what is the greatest factor that can shorten the operation span of a truck. I explain that this would happen if the motor failed. I then compare this to a human whose lifespan is typically sixty years, give or take twenty. Some may die at forty and some at eighty, but somewhere in between this span of time, most people die. I go on to explain that the most common cause of death for humans is cardiovascular disease. This includes damage to our heart, which is our body's motor.

The two trucks traveling the same distance at the same speed for multiple years can be affected if one of the trucks carries a lighter load, such as cardboard, as opposed to the other truck carrying a heavier load like bricks. The truck carrying bricks will have more wear and tear on its motor and other parts. This truck is less likely to continue for eight years as opposed to the truck carrying the cardboard. The same concept applies to humans. If we have undiagnosed, untreated high blood pressure, this causes unnecessary stress on our heart over the years. A person with elevated blood pressure is much more likely to suffer an uneventful heart attack or stroke, which can be fatal. The person with untreated high blood pressure is less likely to live for eighty years. That is why it is so important to have your blood pressure checked, and if it is elevated, comply with a treatment regimen prescribed by your medical provider. The bottom line is, we do have a great deal of control.

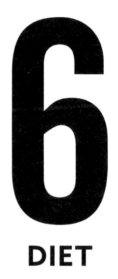

CHAPTER

6

DIET

"**A GOOD DIET INVOLVES MAKING PERSISTENT,** CONSCIOUS DECISIONS ABOUT EVERY FOOD SELECTION BUT REALIZING **THAT IT'S OKAY NOT TO BE PERFECT**."

BLUEPRINT: THE BEST DIET

Mr. and Mrs. Smith were both fifty-five years old, and had been married since college. They wanted to know how to eat healthier. I asked them to imagine a scenario involving an old college friend asking if his daughter, who just got accepted to a residency program, could stay at their home for a couple of weeks while her apartment was being prepared. I looked at Mrs. Smith and told her that the young lady was very beautiful and had a great figure. I then asked Mrs. Smith to imagine her husband going into the kitchen at night for water, and finding the young house guest in the kitchen, not properly dressed. I asked Mrs. Smith how she would feel about this. She replied that the house guest would have to get a hotel room.

I asked the Smiths to compare the young house guest to a bag of chips or cookies in the cabinet. I reassured Mrs. Smith that Mr. Smith would not go for the young lady, but she agreed that this was an unnecessary, unwelcome temptation. I told her that those cookies and chips should also be removed from the home. I encouraged them to remove any tempting foods that would make it difficult for them to eat as healthy as possible.

I informed them of how I had to change the people around me when I was in medical school. Initially, I explained, I would hang out with my fraternity brothers in the nearby undergraduate college. On a Friday, we would talk about the frat party or the Greek show. This would make it impossible to imagine studying on a Friday night, and hard to make it to the study session on a Saturday morning. After my academic advisor suggested I make new friends due to my less-than-optimal grades, I started hanging out with medical students. Almost immediately, I became more successful in my academic performance. The new friends would not talk about the parties but talk about the gross anatomy test on Monday. Support is a huge factor when you are trying to accomplish something as difficult a healthier lifestyle with a better diet. Just as encouragement to study from people that were studying was useful, encouragement to eat healthier by people eating healthy can be beneficial. I encourage patients trying to eat healthy to seek out others doing the same. This way, they may hear about the newest salad bar or smoothie shop in town versus the latest buffet or dessert bar.

What is the best diet? When asked this question last week, I asked the patient if we could play a quiz game. After she agreed, I explained the rules, which included her answering "healthy" or "unhealthy" to food selections presented. I first listed fried chicken dinner or a vegetable plate. She answered with unhealthy to the first and healthy to the second. I then gave a scenario of a friend's daughter in the break room at her place of employment, eating cookies. I expand on this scenario where she accepts three cookies after the little girl offers, and another scenario where she accepts only one cookie. She answers the quiz with the first scenario being less healthy than the first. I informed the patient that she passed the quiz with flying colors. I further explained that we are aware when we eat unhealthy in most cases. I told the patient that we are not going to be perfect, but we must always consider the healthy assessment every time we make a food selection. Like the scenario where the lady only took one cookie, she was better off than taking three. Moderation is not a nasty word. This is especially true when someone is trying to start a healthier lifestyle. I told my patient that a good diet is one that includes making persistent, conscious decisions about every food selection, and realizing that it is ok not to be perfect. A diet written on paper with a structured regimented food selection was unrealistic for a long-term change. In reality, people have different tastes and likes, and can easily become tired of a strict diet regimen. I told her that she could make better choices realistically and long-term for the rest of her life.

Now that we have talked about what to eat, we can now talk about how to eat. Many dieters don't realize that this can have just as big an impact on becoming healthier. The diet consists of eating frequent small meals daily. I was first introduced to this dietary concept in the gym by some professional body builders. These athletes had very little body fat, and were able to take in a lot of daily calories. This same dietary concept is used for the most popular diets including Jenny Craig, Weight Watchers, and The Optifast diet. They did not starve themselves as suggested in many other diets. Many of my patients have implemented this dietary technique over the last ten years. I have witnessed the improved health for many of these dieters firsthand, resulting in better blood pressures and diabetic control. Many patients who were on multiple medications have had their medications reduced, and some have been taken off all their medication over time, in a coordinated process with monitoring.

This dietary technique, which I refer to as the "Q diet" for my patients, has helped me personally. Many of my patients have voiced concerns that they don't have time to eat with this frequency. I explain to them that it is not hard once you develop a routine and include food options readily available. I use supplemental shakes during the day when I am unable to get a break. I drink the shake between patients, while charting notes. Yesterday, I explained to a patient who works on an assembly line that she could have the shake or a breakfast bar in her purse, and eat it on a restroom break. I told her that she did not have to take a lunch break to eat. The most important thing is to provide your body with persistent calories throughout the day.

While doing my residency in Los Angeles, I was introduced to a diet program at UCLA. I was introduced to research in this program and others. This persistent dietary concept was studied with consistent successful results. One study included two groups that both consumed 1,500 calories a day. One group consumed 300 calories five times a day, and the other group consumed 750 calories twice a day. The group that ate more frequent meals lost the most weight, even though both groups ate the same amount of food each day. The group that had the more frequent meals reported less hunger, which helped them not eat food selections not in the diet program.

The body responds to stressors in the environment without our conscious awareness. If we are exposed to extreme prolonged heat, we sweat. If we are exposed to sudden darkness, our pupils will dilate. These changes are controlled automatically by our autonomic nervous system. These changes occur to allow us to survive better. The sweating in the heat is to help us cool down. The dilation of the pupils allows us to see in the dark.

When we skip breakfast or lunch, we have gone a long time between meals. A patient told me last week that he skipped breakfast and lunch most days, but did not lose weight. He told me that he would eat dinner at 7 pm and have lunch at 12 noon. I explained that 12 hours passed from his last meal at 7 pm the night before till 7 the next morning. I further explained that another 5 hours would pass before 12 noon if this was the time he ate lunch after skipping breakfast. I explained that his body would enter starvation mode by allowing 17 hours to pass with no nutrition. I further explained that this was worse if he skipped lunch.

Our autonomic nervous system causes three changes when we skip meals, and put our bodies into the starvation mode. The first change is slowing our metabolic rate down. The body is attempting to hold on to calories, and slows down the metabolism to conserve the calories during long period with no nutrition. Our metabolism automatically slows down as we age. I remember when I was in my twenties and could eat whatever I wanted. I could eat fast food and not gain weight. If I now even look at a fast food restaurant, I gain ten pounds. Eating frequent meals speed up our metabolism. The second change includes less fat storage by eating frequent meals. The body has less need to store excess fat when it realizes that the person is not going to starve the body. Fat has approximately nine calories per gram, which is efficient energy storage as opposed to protein and carbohydrates that only have approximately four calories per gram. The third change is that the person who eats frequent meals has less hunger. By eating frequent meals, the body releases less hunger biochemical into the bloodstream, causing the person to not choose unhealthy snacks like chips or cookies kept in the break room, that are waiting for the opportunity to destroy your new, healthier dietary lifestyle. Many patients have told me that eating small frequent meals helped them have better control. Some admitted to eating cookies at times, but were able to eat one as opposed to the entire container, as they were more likely to do in the past. I explained that this was healthier, and definitely a move in the right direction.

A typical day in my dietary life starts out with me having breakfast no more than thirty minutes after awakening. This usually consists of oatmeal and a veggie link or eggs and grits. I usually have this meal around 7:30 AM. Around 10:30AM, I have my pre-lunch snack. This will usually be a protein shake or a cereal bar. Around 1:30 PM, I have my lunch, which is usually half a sandwich or a bowl of vegetables with a small chicken breast. Around 4:30 PM, I will have the second snack. If I had half a sandwich at lunch, I would eat the other half at this time. I usually have a protein bar or another protein shake, in preparation to go to the gym. My last meal is around 7:30 PM. For this meal, I will have a light dinner, which can vary from a salad with chicken breast or veggies with fish. I keep the portions small. Before going to bed, I usually have fruit to avoid late-night hunger. Notice that I used the term "around" a lot to illustrate that the time does not have to be exact.

For those who are beginners with this new dietary technique, I advise keeping a diary. Writing down food selections and the times of eating help to maintain accountability and increases success. I also advise sharing your diary with a friend or family member, which helps. Studies have repeatedly demonstrated that accountability helps. I had a patient who told me that she felt bad eating the cookie, because she knew she had to turn in her diary to me for review. I laughed when the entry in the food diary read: 6:23 PM - one bite of a cookie. She admitted she probably would have had three cookies, if it were not for the diary.

CHAPTER

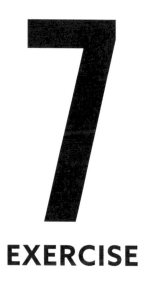

EXERCISE

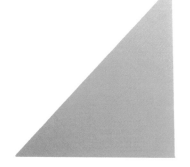

"EXERCISE DOES NOT HAVE TO BE **DREADFUL** BUT CAN REALLY **BE ENJOYABLE."**

BLUEPRINT: EXERCISE

Weight loss results when the output calories are greater than the input. We expend calories through our normal metabolic processes. This includes breathing, our heart beating, eating, thinking, standing or sitting, and other persistent functions of living. These bodily functions are performed automatically. If we desire to expend additional calories, we must increase our activity level. The most effective way to accomplish this is with exercise. I talk with my patients about various exercise options. I inform them that the most effective exercise is one that they can continue long-term.

Mr. Jones was a forty-year-old truck driver and was very overweight. He had poorly controlled diabetes, hypertension, and elevated cholesterol. I explained to him that he would develop complications that could be potentially deadly if we did not get his medical conditions under better control. He refused the option of insulin for the treatment of his diabetes since the insulin would disqualify him for his livelihood as a truck driver. He agreed to implement an exercise and diet regimen as an adjunct to his therapy. He voiced understanding of the dietary concept of the Q diet—the dietary concept described in the previous chapter—but stated that the exercise component would be difficult with his busy schedule and lack of access to a gym. Together, we came up with a strategic plan for an exercise program that fitted his work schedule. He confirmed that the trucks are monitored via satellite to limit the hours of driving daily. He also confirmed that he would at times get tired after driving for many hours without a break. The time restraints on the road and the fatigue resulted in him parking his truck at rest stations on the side of the highway on a regular basis. His exercise regimen included a thirty-minute jog or brisk walk while at the rest stations, two times a day. His first thought, which he shared with me, was his concern that other drivers would think he was crazy. I told him that he was the smartest driver if he followed this plan. On a return visit three months later and sixteen pounds lighter, all his chronic conditions were better controlled. I proudly informed him that the insulin suggestion was now off the table. He laughed as I asked him, "Who is winning now?"

Note that Mr. Jones incorporated a positive lifestyle change with good results. I often explain to my daughter that we have so much control on the outcome of every aspect of our lives. We only have to make the conscious decision that we will make the necessary sacrifices and practice delayed gratification. Mr. Jones told me how he resisted the usual fried chicken, burgers, and fries at the truck stops. He told me how badly he craved the delicious foods, but he maintained his new dietary changes in addition to his exercise regimen. He told me it was not fun, but he implemented changes that made it more pleasant. He purchased a headphone set that he used with his cellphone to listen to his favorite music while he did his workouts. He informed that this helped a lot, because he found himself stepping to the beat as if he were dancing while exercising. He told me that he initially got strange stares, but after his persistence, he started noticing other truck drivers walking and jogging at rest stops. He noted that the number was not great, but some were actually exercising!

You must first find some form of physical activity that you enjoy. Exercise does not have to be dreadful; it can be enjoyable. I am a runner. I have been a runner for long as I can remember. I ran the mile race on the track team in high school, and ran further distances in the military after graduating. I ran while in college and medical school. I remember some of my classmates in medical school picking on me at times, calling me Forest Gump due to my running and being from the south. I get a great deal of enjoyment from running. There have been periods when I have suffered minor injuries, causing me to take breaks for weeks or months at a time. I tried to find other forms of cardiovascular exercise, including swimming and biking. I did not achieve the same level of enjoyment that I achieved with running. I have friends and patients who have other forms of exercise they enjoy. I have one patient who participates in line dancing aerobics, which is a form of cardiovascular exercise involving a dancing routine with popular music. If you enjoy swimming, walking, biking, traditional aerobics or dance aerobics, find your favorite exercise activities. This will ensure a much better chance that you will be able to maintain the persistence required to be truly successful. For some, I suggest consider alternating more than one form of exercise. I alternate weight lifting for two consecutive days for every day of running. This allows rest for the muscles concentrated on, and reduces injuries.

Another way to help with success is to participate in group exercise activities. I usually run alone, but when I lift weights, I prefer to go to a gym with other weightlifters. It is the same scenario like my medical school. I initially studied alone in my apartment, but found myself distracted by the television, telephone, visitors, and other distractions. When I started going to the library to study, after being advised by my academic advisor, I noticed I got a lot more done with fewer distractions. I also noticed that I was influenced by all the other people studying. I remember many Friday and Saturday nights of me planning to get a few hours of studying in at the library before meeting up with friends at a party. On many of these nights, I would find myself watching other medical students studying hard, with no sign of stopping on a Friday or Saturday night. As a result of what I was observing, I would find myself staying in the library till closing time at midnight, and returning at eight the next morning to meet my classmates. This is also the case when I work out at the gym. I may go in with plans for a quick light workout, but end up working out longer and harder due to others working out with increased intensity. I highly recommend group workouts for beginners since persistent motivation can be a factor. Working out with a group, such as an aerobics class or line dancing class, will definitely help you have the accountability you need to be successful. Music is also a way to enhance a workout. I use headphones and listen to my favorite high-intensity music. My mother listens to upbeat gospel music. I advise listening to whatever your favorite music is, and enjoying your exercise sessions.

CHAPTER

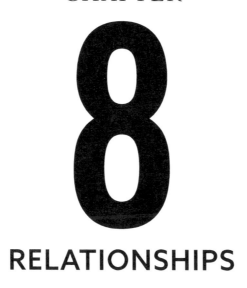

8

RELATIONSHIPS

"I ASSURED HER THAT SHE COULD BE
THE HAPPY LOVER AGAIN WHO WAS IN
THE PICTURE,
BUT SHE MUST BE WILLING TO
UNDERSTAND THAT SHE IS THE ONLY ONE
FULLY IN CONTROL OF CHANGE HERSELF."

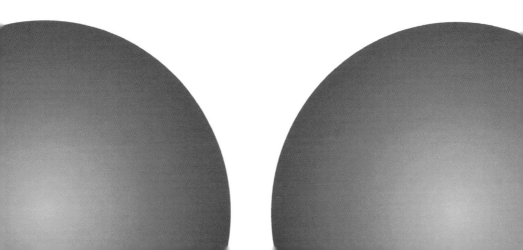

BLUEPRINT: RELATIONSHIPS

Cynthia was a thirty-year-old schoolteacher. Her chief complaint was that she felt sad. After a history confirmed that she was not clinically depressed, I asked specifics of why she felt the way she did. She told me that she had been dating a young man for the last three years, and like her previous relationship of four years, there was no hint of a ring. She told me that she felt that she would make a perfect wife and mother, and dreamed of marriage with children every day. Cynthia told me that she was confused why all her friends were married, but her day seemed like it was not going to come.

I explained to Cynthia that there are many factors to consider when determining why her day has not come. I further explained to her that a large percentage of the problem is beyond her control. I told her to focus on what she could control, and the rest will work itself out. I told her that she had a lot to offer by being educated, attractive, and having a great personality. I also told her that she must realize that she can't control another person.

I told Cynthia that it is important to take a close look at the person she is with, and try to find out what is on his mind. I explained that the man must *want* to be married in order to ask her. A lot of relationships are not clear, and a big part of this is because the discussions that should take place are not happening. A lot of this is fear of thinking that they may receive information they don't want to hear. Another fear is that the person being asked the questions will feel pressured. I highly encourage anyone in a relationship to have a discussion with their partner to ensure they are going in the same direction.

I also encourage people in a relationship to not only listen to what is said, but pay closer attention to what is done. I told Cynthia about a previous relationship involving my girlfriend and myself coming out of a Wal-Mart. She was on the outside, exposed to oncoming cars. I found myself, without even realizing, repositioning myself on the outside so she was protected from oncoming cars. I noticed what I had done when she smiled as she put her arm around me. I realized, at that moment, that I cared for her in a way that let me know we were headed toward a long-term relationship if she so desired. The reason I told that story was to inform that I was not even aware of how I felt at that time. The bottom line is that men, such as myself, sometimes have a hard time understanding what we feel. We certainly have a very difficult time articulating how we feel. This is why it is so important that ladies watch what we do to a greater degree, compared to what we say. Other examples of men considering the lady above our personal desires can include: watching a reality show with our lady over Monday night football, going to church with our lady over sleeping in, taking our lady on a romantic date over watching television every Saturday night at her house, spending quality time with our lady over hanging with our boys, and other signs to include phone calls or texts for no reason to say nothing more than we were thinking of you.

I further encouraged Cynthia to have that discussion with her boyfriend, and pay close attention to the signs. I added that she makes the decision about their future based on her findings, and not have regrets. I also encouraged her to not be in such a rush to get any guy, but take her time to ensure she chooses the right guy. I ended the session by telling Cynthia that it is ok to be alone sometimes.

The person in the mirror can be your best friend and your worst enemy. One of the most wonderful gifts of life is the ability to choose. We have far more power over our life than we realize, and gaining an understanding of the significant impact our decisions can have on our lives, can make all the difference in the world. I have heard many people say that they wish they knew in the past what they know now. As we age, we make better decisions due to a better understanding of consequences of those decisions. Some of the consequences are good, and some not so good. Early in life, I learned to look in the mirror and see the person responsible for most of my life's outcomes. I am aware that some things are uncontrollable, but I also understand that exhausting every resource will give me the best chance of a more favorable outcome in these uncontrollable situations.

Miss Jones was a thirty-two-year-old teacher who came in with the chief complaint of fatigue. I remember my first impression upon entering the exam room. I saw an angry, frustrated lady who appeared very unhappy. Her first statement to me was that she was going through a divorce. My response was, "My name is Dr. Quinn, and it is a pleasure to meet you." I think I detected a fraction of a smile to meet my big smile as I made the statement. As Miss Jones talked about her situation, I noticed that she blamed many people and circumstances. She gave the classic impression of someone with the "victim mentality."

After we reviewed her initial lab work and determined that it was unlikely she had a medical condition causing her to feel tired, I asked if I could help her find the true solution. Puzzled, she asked what I suggested. I asked her if she wanted her marriage. Miss Jones told me that she wanted it more than anything for herself and their six-year-old daughter. I told her that the strategy starts now. I told her to go home, clean up, cook her husband his favorite meal, and prepare to give him a full body massage after dinner. Her first response was that she was not going to cook him anything, or clean the house, and that she was definitely not going to touch him. She started to repeat how he does not look at her the way he used to. She further explained that he does not talk to her or make her feel beautiful. I asked her if she had a picture of them early in the relationship, before they were married. She showed me a picture on her Facebook page, and as I suspected, I saw a different lady in the picture. I asked her if she would accept an assignment of going home and spending no less than an hour a day for one week looking at the picture. She was then to spend fifteen minutes a day, writing down thoughts and feelings she remembered during the time of the taking of the picture.

The following week, Miss Jones signed in for her follow-up appointment. Upon entering the room, she excitedly told me of her findings. She reported feeling loved during the taking of the picture. She remembered a lot of facts that she happily reported. I stopped her, and asked her to pull the picture up on her phone once again. I pointed out that her disposition in the picture was different from the lady I recently met. I told her that she can be the happy lover in the picture, but she must be willing to understand that the only person she has full control to change is herself. She must take the focus of change from her husband, and accept the responsibility of working on changing herself. I suggested she start with her appearance. I reminded her that she wanted him to see her as beautiful again, but she admitted she had not got her hair or nails done in over a year. She also admitted that she gained forty pounds since the picture due to not exercising and eating healthy since the wedding, which she used to do religiously earlier. I told her that the change in her attitude toward him was more damaging than any other contributing factor. For her to tell me that she would not touch him, and never give him a massage, was telling. She admitted that she speaks in a derogatory fashion to him, and discourages him as opposed to encourage him. She further admitted that this stemmed from his lack of success in a company he started, resulting in her carrying the majority of the financial responsibility of the family. She told me that she was angry with him for being a failure.

After four follow up visits and a lot of counseling, Miss Jones accepted the challenge to focus all her efforts on herself. She understood that Miss Jones was the only one who controlled Miss Jones, and her husband and his success was not hers to control. She also stated that she would do everything in her power to make her situation better. She started with her physical appearance. She worked on her weight, started getting her hair and nails done, and wore nice clothing. She changed her attitude toward her husband. She focused her conversation with him on how she admired him for wanting to start his own company and be a leader. She would tell him how proud she was of him for not being afraid to take risks, and not limit his future like most others. She started helping out with his business, and investing her time and connections.

In less than one year, she came to the office to thank me. She looked great. She was well groomed with a new hairstyle, was thirty pounds lighter, and her smile lit up the room. She told me she had some big news. Miss Jones told me she was still married to the best man on earth whose business is affording them to purchase the new home of her dreams. While she was telling of the wonderful events, she started to cry. With tears in her eyes, she told me that it was confirmed by her OBGYN yesterday that she was two months pregnant. The nurse entered the room to find the both of us with tears of joy.

It is truly amazing how much impact we can have on a situation by just focusing on changing ourselves. The biggest change includes changing our attitude. I have had so many situations that seemed impossible, but were made possible when I realized that changing my attitude was helpful. A perfect example was a professor who did not like me. Some may ask how I reached this conclusion. The man told me that he did not like "my kind." He explained that he felt I did not belong in medical school because "Guys like you don't become doctors." His impression of me was not that of a traditional medical student. I left his office angry with the first thought of "forget him." The word was not actually "forget," but I think you get the picture.

I remember going home angry, but remembering the lessons I had learned. I started by looking into my mirror and acknowledging that this was the only guy I could control. I immediately took the course book and started to outline the next chapter that was to be covered in the next class session with the professor. I then wrote a report on the chapter. When the next class started, I sat in the front after turning the unrequested work in. I took notes, and asked and answered questions. I approached every class session for the remainder of the semester in the same manner. Some of my classmates told me I was kissing up. I told them that I was doing my best. I received a B plus for the class that many failed, and an apology. The professor told me that he was wrong about me, and wrote one of my best letters of recommendation for residency when I graduated.

When you make up your mind that you are going to start with yourself to change your situation, you must not let others distract you. You must stay the course, no matter the outcome. If I would have failed the class, I would have not been disappointed because I knew that I did all I could do. I remember early in our sessions, I told Miss Jones to not be disappointed if her marriage failed, because she was doing all she could. With this attitude, you will not always win the battle, but you will put yourself in the best position to win the war.

CHAPTER

9

PRADER

"I REMEMBER MY GRANDFATHER
TELLING ME THAT
THE BEST WAY TO GIVE GOD PRAISE FOR HIS GRACE
IS TO SHOW THAT YOU APPRECIATE
YOUR EARTHLY GIFTS
AND TO USE THEM."

BLUEPRINT: PRAYER

B y no means do I proclaim to be an expert on religion or faith. Like the rest of this book, I simply illustrate examples from the lives of others and my own with scenarios that are made better by their choice of action. My grandfather was a great minister of the Church of God in Christ. He shared his wisdom with me till his last days. He taught me that we must have faith, and demonstrate our faith by acting.

An example of my grandfather's teachings included a conversation that we had regarding my poor initial performance in medical school. I remember calling my grandfather back in Mississippi, and telling him that he needed to tell God that I needed to pass all the classes so I could graduate. He asked me if I really believed in God, and if I believed that this was God's will. He explained that my gift of retention, which I demonstrated in my undergraduate academic accomplishments, proved that I could handle the work load with hard work and greater dedication, and achieve my desired success. He further explained that it was an unwise prayer to pray for something that God has already blessed me with. After this conversation, I remembered his teachings, and prayed for greater discipline, greater dedication, and motivation. With my new prayer and guidance, I spent more time in the library, and less time worrying. This resulted in my successful graduation from medical school.

Miss Jones is a patient that I often use as an example when lecturing on this topic. She told me that she was in the process of getting kicked out of her apartment, and stood the possibility of losing her children due to the inability to provide appropriately. When asked about her employment, she told me that she was waiting on a job. When asked about her search methods, she told me that she was praying daily, but decided to wait on God. With the greatest respect, I commended her for her faith, but told of my grandfather's teachings. I encouraged her to become more proactive by searching for a job on the internet and seeking immediate employment with a local temporary agency. After I made a call from my office to a temporary agency, she was asked to come in for the job training the next day. On a follow up visit, she informed that she changed her prayer to help her work harder than she ever did before. Miss Jones told me that she prayed that her temporary employer would find favor in her work, and hire her for a permanent position. She told me that she believed that her prayer was answered, because the more she believed, the harder and more effectively she performed. This patient later reported that her faith helped her secure the job she needed to provide for her family.

My grandfather talked about God's favor, and how He loved us. I remember my graduation from medical school being late due to a requirement to take a final board exam after graduation as I hadn't passed the first time around. This delayed the start date of my residency training. In the six-month interim, I took a job as a college professor. I distinctly remember two students. One student was a smart woman and the second was a man who was very challenged academically. The female student would hardly show up for classes, sat in the back, and talked the entire duration of the class, had a bad attitude of entitlement, and turned in only half of her work. The male student never missed a class, sat in the front, stayed after classes to ask questions, and did extra work on all assignments. At the end of the semester, both students were on the verge of passing or failing, and had to turn in a ten-page paper for the final grade. The woman's paper was only seven pages, but brilliantly written. The man's paper was twenty pages, but not well written. One student was shown favor.

I often use this story of the two students when illustrating a point to my audiences about favor. I then ask the listener to imagine a scenario where you or someone you love is asking for God's favor. I ask them to imagine needing that job, getting that passing score, overcoming that medical diagnosis, or any other scenario where you find yourself in prayer. I then remind them of the two students coming to my office the following week, asking for favor to pass the class. I remember the conversations so well. The male reminded me of how hard he worked, and the dedication and persistence he showed. The female student apologized for her lack of hard work, and lack of dedication and persistence. As you probably imagined, the student that passed the class was the male student. I then ask the listener which scenario they would want to give in their prayers. Would you rather tell our Creator that you have done all that you can do by His grace? I remind the listener that we serve a benevolent forgiving God who is ultimately in control. No matter our actions or prayers, He takes the final decision. I then remind the listener of my grandfather's words: "It never hurts to show Him that you are willing to do all you can."

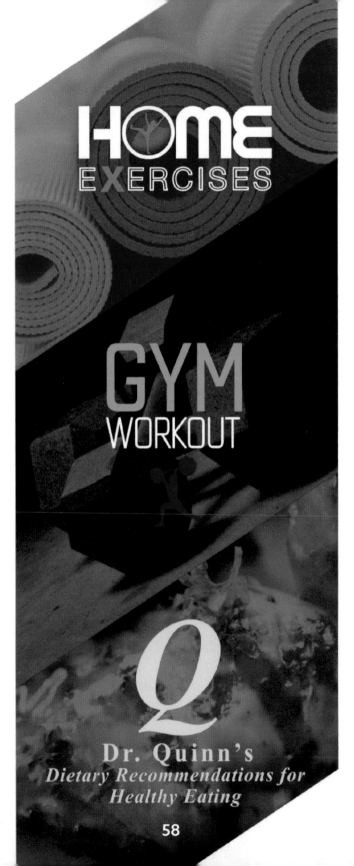

HOME EXERCISES

GYM
WORKOUT

Dr. Quinn's
Dietary Recommendations for Healthy Eating

PLEASE READ

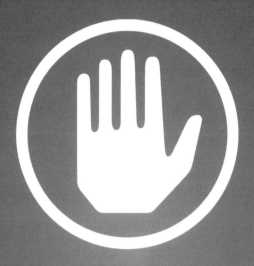

If you are concerned that you feel discomfort
while performing any activity,
stop and call your doctor.

Always use proper technique,
remembering to maintain correct
form with slow and controlled movements.

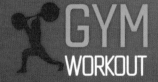 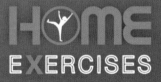

BY: JAMES MARTIN

MS - ACSM Certified Exercise Physiologist &
NASM Certified Personal Trainer
jamart30@hotmail.com | 662.242.0520

HOME
EXERCISES

It is advised to consult with your medical provider prior to starting
an exercise program such as this.
It is also advised to stop exercising immediately
if you have any symptoms of shortness
of breath or chest pain, and not hesitate to seek emergency medical assistance.

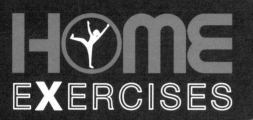

HOME EXERCISES

Beginners Level:
3 Sets Of (1 to 10 Repetitions)
Moderate Level:
3 Sets Of (11 to 15 Repetitions)
Advanced Level: 3
Sets Of (16 or More Repositions)

MONDAY
WEDNESDAY
FRIDAY

Marching

A. Simply march in place by lifting feet (alternating)
B. Maintain correct posture during movement

Many people believe you need a lot of equipment and space to get a quality workout but you don't. Here are the exercises broken down:

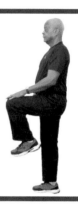

General Stretching

A. Upper Body Stretches
B. Lower Body Stretches
C. Maintain Correct Posture

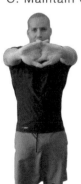
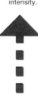
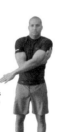
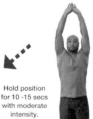

Hold position for 10 -15 secs with moderate intensity.

Hold position for 10 -15 secs with moderate intensity.

Hold position for 10 -15 secs with moderate intensity.

Repeat with opposite arm.

Hold position for 10 -15 secs with moderate intensity.

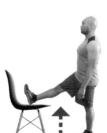
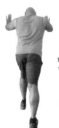

Hold position for 10 -15 secs with moderate intensity.

Repeat with opposite leg.

Hold position for 10 -15 secs with moderate intensity.

Repeat with opposite leg.

61

H✦ME
EXERCISES

Beginners Level
3 Sets Of (1 to 10 Repetitions)
Moderate Level
3 Sets Of (11 to 15 Repetitions)
Advanced Level:
Sets Of (16 or More Repositions)

Front Arm Raises

A. Start with hands by your side
B. Lift Resistance upward and forward to shoulder height
C. Lower the weight to the original position in a slow controlled motion maintaining resistance
D. Maintain proper posture

In the event that you don't have home dumbbell weights, you can substitute with a jug. Fill the jug with water to a level that produces a weight with good resistance.

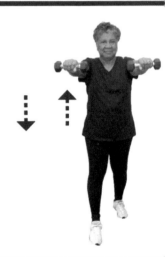

Side Arm Raises

A. Start with hands by your side
B. Lift Resistance upward and forward to shoulder height
C. Lower the weight to the original position in a slow controlled motion maintaining resistance
D. Maintain proper posture

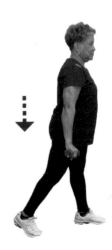
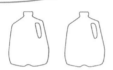

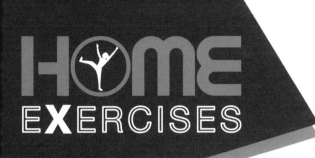

Beginners Level:
3 Sets Of (1 to 10 Repetitions)
Moderate Level:
3 Sets Of (11 to 15 Repetitions)
Advanced Level: 3
Sets Of (16 or More Repositions)

Wall Push Ups

A. Stand facing wall
B. Extend arms to wall
C. Lean body toward wall
D. Push back and repeat

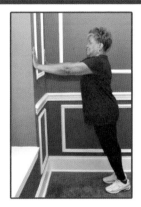 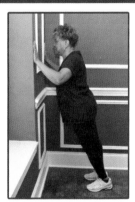

Seated Leg Raises

A. Sit with rib cage lifted up
B. Extend one leg out and hold
C. Alternate leg and repeat

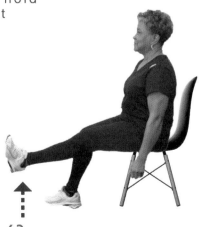

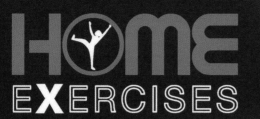

HOME EXERCISES

Beginners Level
3 Sets Of (1 to 10 Repetitions)
Moderate Level
3 Sets Of (11 to 15 Repetitions)
Advanced Level:
Sets Of (16 or More Repositions)

If you do not have an exercise ball you can use a large pillow to replace the ball to perform the exercise as demonstrated.

Overhead Ball Squeeze

A. Lift ball overhead in a slight lunge position
B. Squeeze and hold
C. Lower to the original position in a controlled slow motion to maintain resistance
D. Repeat while maintaining correct posture

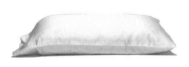

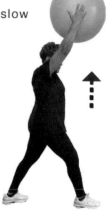

Chair Squats

A. From a seated position
B. Stand making sure knees never go pass toes
C. Repeat

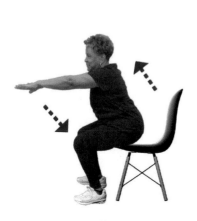

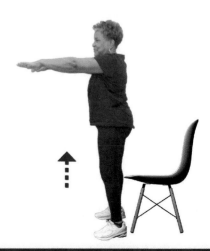

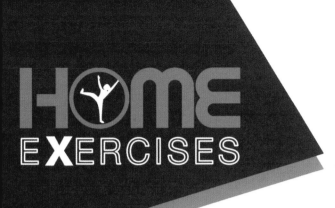

Beginners Level:
3 Sets Of (1 to 10 Repetitions)
Moderate Level:
3 Sets Of (11 to 15 Repetitions)
Advanced Level: 3
Sets Of (16 or More Repositions)

Bent Over Row

A. Slightly bend at waist into a lunge position
B. Keep back straight
C. Place one hand on chair
D. Lift weight upward with other hand

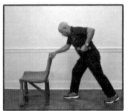
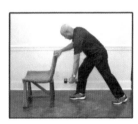

Wall Sits

A. Squat down with back against wall
   with legs bent at a 90' degrees
B. Keep arms by your side with shoulders back
C. Maintain perfect posture
D. Return to standing position and repeat
   the number of suggested repetitions

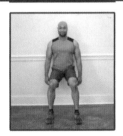

Triceps Kickback

A. From a lunge position place one hand on chair
B. Pull opposite elbow up into a 90' angle
C. Hold elbow in position and extend lower arm backward
D. Return hand to the original position in a control slow motion
   maintaining resistance
E. Repeat this exercise with the opposite hand for the suggested
   number of repetitions

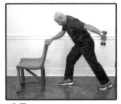
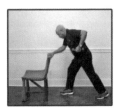

HOME EXERCISES

Beginners Level
3 Sets Of (1 to 10 Repetitions)
Moderate Level
3 Sets Of (11 to 15 Repetitions)
Advanced Level: 3
Sets Of (16 or More Repositions)

Floor Crunches

A. Lie on floor with hand cradling back of head
B. Bend knees keeping feet flat
C. Press lower back into floor
D. Slightly raising shoulder blades

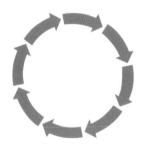
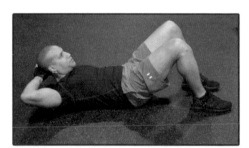

Lower Body Stretches

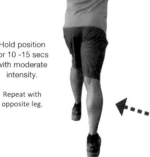
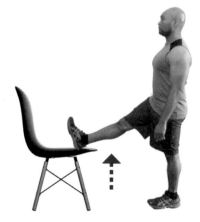

Hold position
for 10 -15 secs
with moderate
intensity.

Repeat with
opposite leg.

Hold position
for 10 -15 secs
with moderate
intensity.

Repeat with
opposite leg.

HOME EXERCISES

TUESDAY — THURSDAY —
WORKOUT

WALK 10 - 30 MINS

General Stretching
A. Upper Body Stretches
B. Lower Body Stretches
C. Maintain Correct Posture

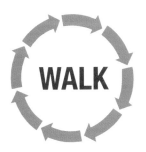

Hold position for 10 -15 secs with moderate intensity.

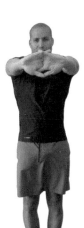

Hold position for 10 -15 secs with moderate intensity.

Hold position for 10 -15 secs with moderate intensity.

Repeat with opposite arm.

Hold position for 10 -15 secs with moderate intensity.

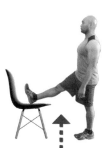

Hold position for 10 -15 secs with moderate intensity.

Repeat with opposite leg.

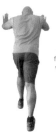

Hold position for 10 -15 secs with moderate intensity.

Repeat with opposite leg.

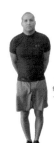
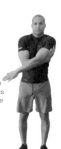
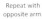

67

Saturday Workout:
Day of Fun with Cardiovascular & Stretching activities.

Sunday Workout:
Day of Rest and Spiritual Growth

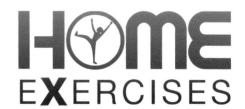

HOME
EXERCISES

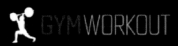

GYM
WORKOUT

It is advised to consult with your medical provider prior to starting an exercise program such as this. It is also advised to stop exercising immediately if you have any symptoms of shortness of breath or chest pain, and not hesitate to seek emergency medical assistance.

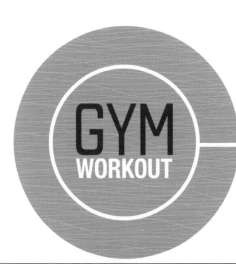

GYM WORKOUT

MONDAY WORKOUT | CHEST & LEG DAY:

(1)

WARM UP!
5-10 MINS

(2) Upper Body Stretches

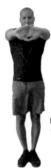 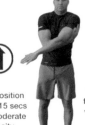 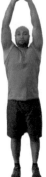 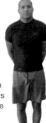

Hold position for 10 -15 secs with moderate intensity.

Hold position for 10 -15 secs with moderate intensity.

Repeat with opposite arm.

Hold position for 10 -15 secs with moderate intensity.

Hold position for 10 -15 secs with moderate intensity.

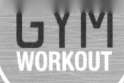

GYM WORKOUT

③ Flat Bench Press
(3 sets X 12 Repetitions)

④ Incline Dumbbell Press
(3 sets X 12 Repetitions)

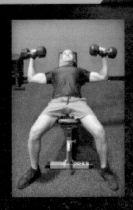
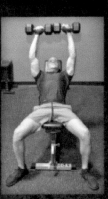

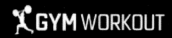

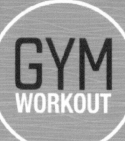

GYM WORKOUT

(5) Push – Ups [3 sets X 20]

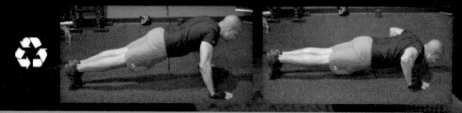

(6) Long Bar Squats [3 sets X 12 Repetitions]

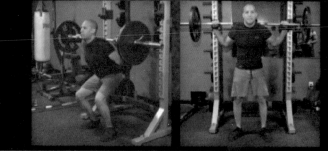

(7) Seated Leg Extensions [3 sets X 12 Repetitions]

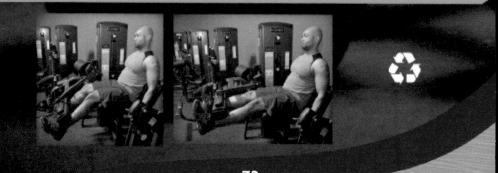

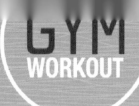
(8) Seated Leg Curls [3 sets X 12 Repetitions]

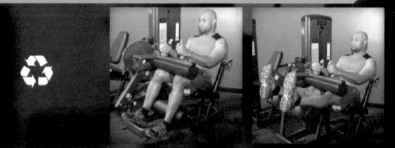

(9) Seated Calf Raises [3 sets X 12 Repetitions]

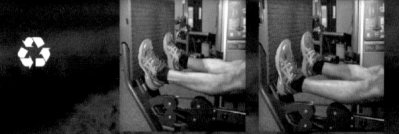

(10) Abdominal Crunches [3 sets X 30 Repetitions]

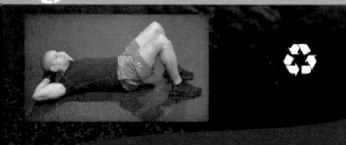

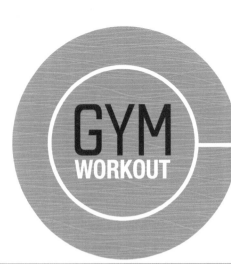

(11) Lower Body Stretches

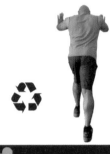

Hold position for 10 -15 secs with moderate intensity.

Repeat with opposite leg.

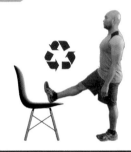

Hold position for 10 -15 secs with moderate intensity.

Repeat with opposite leg.

🏋 TUESDAY WORKOUT | CARDIOVASCULAR & STRETCH DAY :

Cardiovascular Workout:
30 to 60 minutes of walking, biking, treadmill, elliptical machine, swimming, and/or any other form of aerobic exercise that's enjoyable and tolerable.

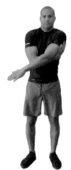

Hold position for 10 -15 secs with moderate intensity.

Repeat with opposite leg.

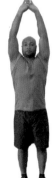

Hold position for 10 -15 secs with moderate intensity.

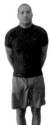

Hold position for 10 -15 secs with moderate intensity.

Hold position for 10 -15 secs with moderate intensity.

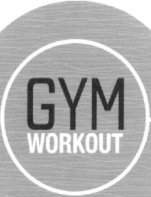

GYM WORKOUT

WEDNESDAY WORKOUT | SHOULDER & TRICEP DAY :

① WARM UP! 5-10 MINS

② Upper Body Stretches

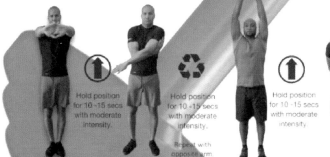

Hold position for 10 -15 secs with moderate intensity.

Hold position for 10 -15 secs with moderate intensity. Repeat with opposite arm.

Hold position for 10 -15 secs with moderate intensity.

Hold position for 10 -15 secs with moderate intensity.

③ Seated Dumbbells Shoulder Press
(3 sets X 12 Repetitions)

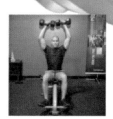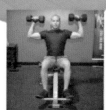

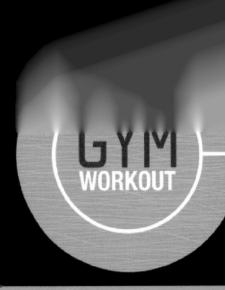

GYM
WORKOUT

4 **Lateral Dumbbell Shoulder Raises**
[3 sets X 12 Repetitions]

5 **Front Dumbbell Shoulder Raises**
[3 sets X 12 Repetitions]

6 **Bent Over Tricep Kickbacks**
[3 sets X 12 Repetitions]

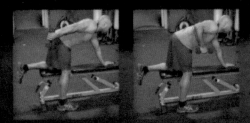

Repeat with
opposite arm.

GYM
WORKOUT

(7) Seated Tricep Press
(3 sets X 12 Repetitions)

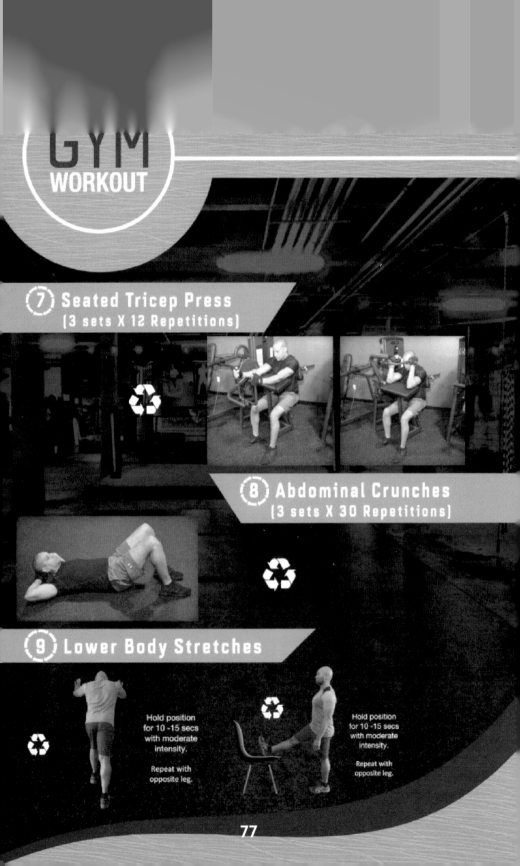

(8) Abdominal Crunches
(3 sets X 30 Repetitions)

(9) Lower Body Stretches

Hold position
for 10 -15 secs
with moderate
intensity.

Repeat with
opposite leg.

Hold position
for 10 -15 secs
with moderate
intensity.

Repeat with
opposite leg.

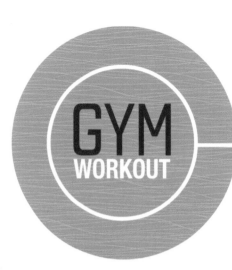

🏋️ THURSDAY WORKOUT | CARDIOVASCULAR & STRETCH DAY

Cardiovascular Workout:
30 to 60 minutes of walking, biking, treadmill, elliptical machine, swimming, and/or any other form of aerobic exercise that's enjoyable and tolerable.

Upper Body

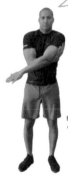

Hold position for 10 -15 secs with moderate intensity.

Repeat with opposite arm

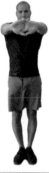

Hold position for 10 -15 secs with moderate intensity.

Hold position for 10 -15 secs with moderate intensity.

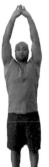

Hold position for 10 -15 secs with moderate intensity.

(11) Lower Body Stretches

Lower Body

Hold position for 10 -15 secs with moderate intensity.

Repeat with opposite leg.

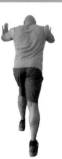

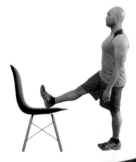

Hold position for 10 -15 secs with moderate intensity.

Repeat with opposite leg.

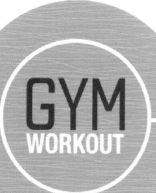

FRIDAY WORKOUT | BACK & BICEP DAY :

(1) WARM UP! 5-10 MINS

(2) Upper Body Stretches

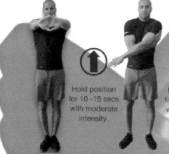

Hold position for 10 -15 secs with moderate intensity.

Hold position for 10 -15 secs with moderate intensity.

Repeat with opposite arm

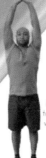

Hold position for 10 -15 secs with moderate intensity.

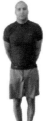

Hold position for 10 -15 secs with moderate intensity.

(3) Pull Ups (3 sets X 8 Repetitions)

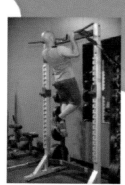

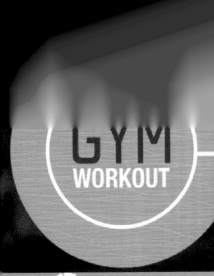

GYM
WORKOUT

(4) Bench Bent Over Row [3 sets X 12 Repetitions]

Repeat with
opposite arm.

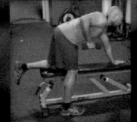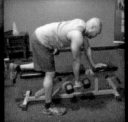

(5) Seated Machine Pulldowns
[3 sets X 12 Repetitions]

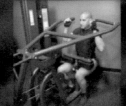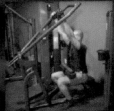

(6) Curl Bar Arm Curls [3 sets X 12 Repetitions]

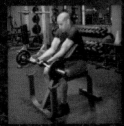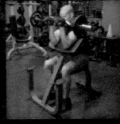

GYM
WORKOUT

(7) Dumbbell Curls (3 sets X 10 Repetitions)

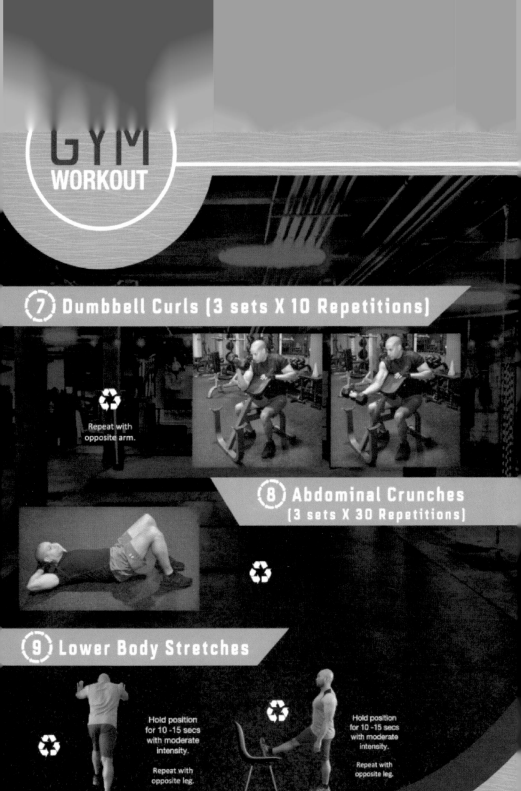

Repeat with opposite arm.

(8) Abdominal Crunches (3 sets X 30 Repetitions)

(9) Lower Body Stretches

Hold position for 10 -15 secs with moderate intensity.

Repeat with opposite leg.

Hold position for 10 -15 secs with moderate intensity.

Repeat with opposite leg.

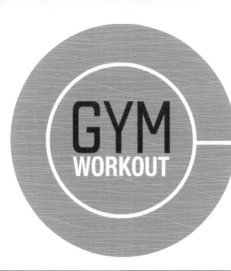

SATURDAY WORKOUT | CARDIOVASCULAR & STRETCH DAY:

Cardiovascular Workout:
30 to 60 minutes of walking, biking, treadmill, elliptical machine, swimming, and/or any other form of aerobic exercise that's enjoyable and tolerable.

Upper Body

Hold position
for 10 -15 secs
with moderate
intensity.

Repeat with
opposite arm

Hold position
for 10 -15 secs
with moderate
intensity.

Hold position
for 10 -15 secs
with moderate
intensity.

Hold position
for 10 -15 secs
with moderate
intensity.

(11) Lower Body Stretches

Lower Body

Hold position
for 10 -15 secs
with moderate
intensity.

Repeat with
opposite leg.

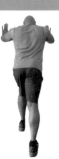

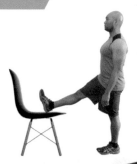

Hold position
for 10 -15 secs
with moderate
intensity.

Repeat with
opposite leg.

SUNDAY
WORKOUT
DAY OF REST
&
SPIRITUAL GROWTH

GYM WORKOUT

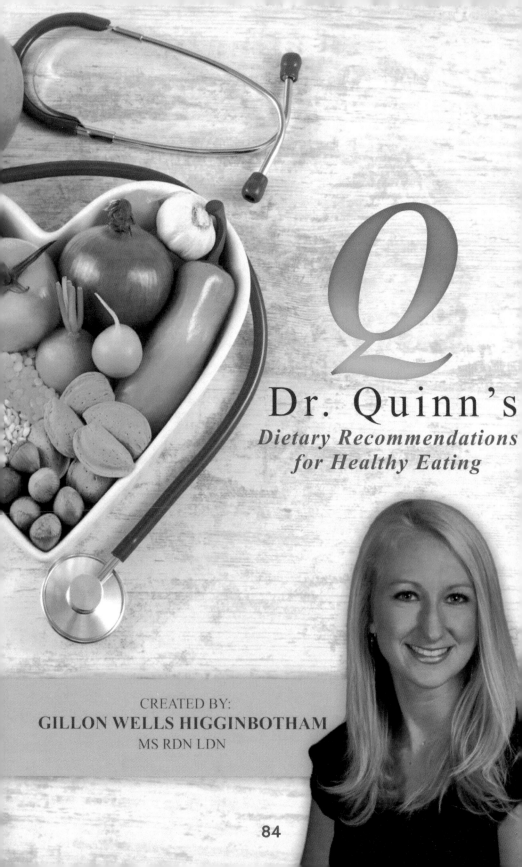

Dr. Quinn's
Dietary Recommendations for Healthy Eating

CREATED BY:

GILLON WELLS HIGGINBOTHAM

MS RDN LDN

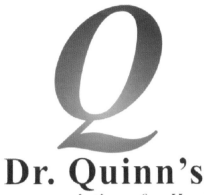

Dr. Quinn's

Dietary Recommendations for Healthy Eating

Created by Gillon Wells Higginbotham MS RDN LDN

Dr. Quinn's healthy eating concept is simple: eat approximately every three hours to maintain energy and minimize hunger, and cravings. The three sample menus below are excellent examples of how the diet strategy works. You can choose from three calorie ranges:

1500 to 1600 calories

1800 to 1900 calories

2000 to 2200 calories.

Portion sizes vary between menus related to the differences in calories. Each menu contains five days of meal and snack options. A good rule of thumb is to try to keep meals less than 500 calories and snacks less than 300 calories. Don't forget to stay hydrated by drinking water throughout the day. The menus provided are tools designed to provide you a road map for healthy eating. You can substitute the meals and snacks for different days of the week based on your individual preference.

What do you do on weekends? Staying in your new routine of eating approximately every three hours – even on weekends - is important. Also, it is okay to occasionally treat yourself to a special meal or dessert with family or friends. If you plan to splurge one evening during dinner, remember to consume smaller meals and snacks throughout the day before dinner. Be creative when planning your meals during the week and weekend. Adding new vegetables, fruits, proteins, and grains to your meals, trying new recipes, and experimenting with new cooking methods are all part of the fun of healthy eating. Choosing healthy meals and snacks can lead to a healthier you.

Check out the helpful tips following the sample menus for ideas on how to eat healthy away from home and when you are traveling.

Meal Plan Tips

Practice Mindful Eating and plan ahead.
Write down ideas for meal options and snacks before going to the grocery store. Choose a variety of fruit,
vegetables, grains, and protein sources.
Make your plate colorful.
Be creative. Trying new recipes and cooking methods can be fun. Healthy cooking methods include baking,
boiling, broiling, grilling, or steaming. Store leftovers for a meal the next day.

Healthy Snack Tips

Keep snacks less than 200 to 300 calories.
For a lighter snack, keep snacks between 100 to 200 calories.
Snacks less than 140mg sodium.
Snacks less than 2gm of saturated fat.
Choose snacks high in fiber to keep you fuller longer.
Snacks with carbohydrates, protein, and fat are great choices.
Check out the nutrition facts food label to help make better choices.
Decrease "empty calorie" foods such as ice cream, soda, candy, cookies, and energy drinks. Try a snack bar
or snack shake that is less than 300 calories, less than 2gm saturated fat.

Grocery Shopping Tips

Plan ahead and make a list.
Decrease temptations by having a snack before going to the store. Select fruits and vegetables that are in
season for cost savings. Check out the grocery store ad for coupons and specials. Select canned vegetables
and soups with lower salt or no salt added. Select canned fruits in water or 100% juice.
Try frozen fresh vegetables and fruits for a change

Avoid aisles with highly processed meals and snack foods.

Reading Nutrition Facts Lables

Review and compare the serving size and servings per container. Review total calories, fat, sodium,
carbohydrates, and protein. Total carbohydrates include fiber and sugar.

Tips for Eating on The Go or Away from Home

Plan ahead before leaving the house.
Pack snacks and water in a cooler for your next road trip.
Limit foods with descriptions such as "Fried, Breaded, or Sautéed with garlic, butter, cream sauce." For
larger restaurant chains, check out the website for nutrition facts to help make healthier choices. Share
large entrees or desserts with a friend.
Ask for a to go box and save some for later.

Nutrient values are subject to change depending on brand, serving size, and cooking method.
Common abbreviations: CHO-Carbohydrate, PRO-Protein, gm.-Gram, Tbsp.-Tablespoon, tsp. - Teaspoon, oz.-Ounce

Sources:
American Diabetes Association & Academy of Nutrition and Dietetics. (2014). Choose your foods: Food lists for Diabetes. United Stat
Department of Agriculture. (2017). USDA food composition databases. Retrieved from https://ndb.nal.usda.gov/ndb/

1 DAY

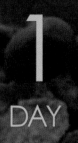

Dr. Quinn's
Dietary Recommendations for Healthy Eating

BREAKFAST

¾ Cup Cereal, Un-sweetened	100 Calories, 22gm CHO, 1gm FAT, 2gm PRO
1 Egg, Hardboiled	70 Calories, 0gm CHO, 5gm FAT, 6gm PRO
1 Cup Skim Milk	80 Calories, 12gm CHO, 0gm FAT, 8gm PRO
1 Cup Coffee	2 Calories, 0gm CHO, 0gm FAT, 0gm PRO

Snack

1 Small Banana	90 Calories, 23gm CHO, 0gm FAT, 1gm PRO
2 Tbsp. Peanut Butter	190 Calories, 8gm CHO, 16gm FAT, 7gm PRO

LUNCH

1 Cup Low Sodium Tomato Soup	75 Calories, 16gm CHO, 1gm FAT, 2gm PRO
4 to 6 Crackers	90 Calories, 9gm CHO, 5gm FAT, 1gm PRO
2 Cups Mixed Green Salad	50 Calories, 10gm CHO, 0gm FAT, 2gm PRO
2 Tbsp. Light Ranch Dressing	80 Calories, 3gm CHO, 7gm FAT, 1gm PRO

Snack

1 oz. Mixed Nuts	170 Calories, 6gm CHO, 15gm FAT, 6gm PRO

MENU 1

1500 - 1600 Calories
(Moderately Overweight Females)

1
DAY

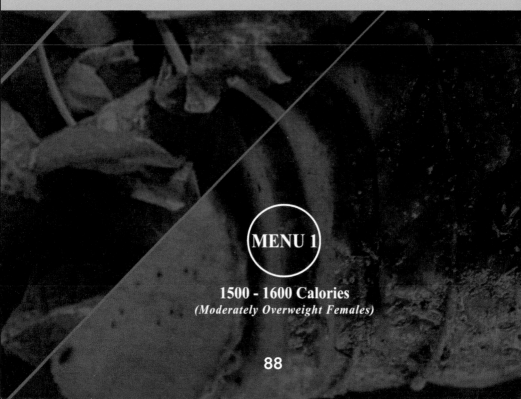DINNER

3 oz. Pork Loin, Baked	165 Calories, 0gm CHO, 2gm FAT, 17gm PR(
1 Cup (~10) Brussels Sprouts (Baked)	90 Calories, 15gm CHO, 0gm FAT, 6gm PRO
1/2 Cup Black-Eyed Peas	90 Calories, 15gm CHO, 1gm FAT, 5gm PRO
1 Small Dinner Roll	80 Calories, 15gm CHO, 1gm FAT, 3gm PRO

Snack

1 Cup Nonfat Flavored Yogurt	120 Calories, 19gm CHO, 0gm FAT, 12gm PRO
1/2 Cup Strawberries, Sliced	30 Calories, 7gm CHO, 0gm FAT, 1gm PRO

MENU 1

1500 - 1600 Calories
(Moderately Overweight Females)

2 DAY

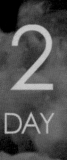

Q
Dr. Quinn's
Dietary Recommendations for Healthy Eating

BREAKFAST

1 Cup Oatmeal, Cooked	150 Calories, 27gm CHO, 2gm FAT, 5gm PRO
1/ 2 Cup Fresh or Frozen Blueberries	42 Calories, 11gm CHO, 0gm FAT, 1gm PRO
1 Vegetable Breakfast Sausage	80 Calories, 3gm CHO, 3gm FAT, 10gm PRO
1 Cup Skim Milk	80 Calories, 12gm CHO, 0gm FAT, 8gm PRO
1 Cup Coffee	2 Calories, 0gm CHO, 0gm FAT, 0gm PRO

Snack

4 to 6 Crackers	90 Calories, 9gm CHO, 5gm FAT, 1gm PRO
1 Mozzarella String Cheese	80 Calories, 0gm CHO, 6gm FAT, 7gm PRO

LUNCH

1 Chicken Wrap With Fresh Vegetables

1 Whole Wheat Tortilla Wrap	130 Calories, 22gm CHO, 3gm FAT, 3gm PRO
3 oz. Chicken Breast, Chopped	105 Calories, 0gm CHO, 4gm FAT, 16gm PRO
1/2 Cup Mixed Vegetables, Roasted	25 Calories, 5gm CHO, 0gm FAT, 1gm PRO
2 Tbsp. Light Ranch Dressing	80 Calories, 3gm CHO, 7gm FAT, 1gm PRO

Snack

1 Cup Nonfat Flavored Yogurt	120 Calories, 19gm CHO, 0gm FAT, 12gm PRO
2 Tbsp. Granola	60 Calories, 10gm CHO, 2gm FAT, 1gm PRO

MENU 1

1500 - 1600 Calories
(Moderately Overweight Females)

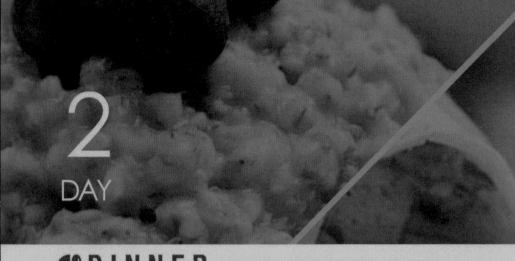

2
DAY

🍴DINNER

3 oz. Salmon, Baked	130 Calories, 0gm CHO, 5gm FAT, 21gm PRO
½ Cup Red Potato Wedges, Baked	80 Calories, 15gm CHO, 0gm FAT, 3gm PRO
2 Cups Mixed Green Salad	50 Calories, 10gm CHO, 0gm FAT, 2gm PRO
2 Tbsp. Light Italian Dressing	35 Calories, 3gm CHO, 3gm FAT, 0gm PRO

Snack

1 Medium Apple	80 Calories, 22gm CHO, 0gm FAT, 0gm PRO
1 Tbsp. Peanut Butter	95 Calories, 4gm CHO, 8gm FAT, 4gm PRO

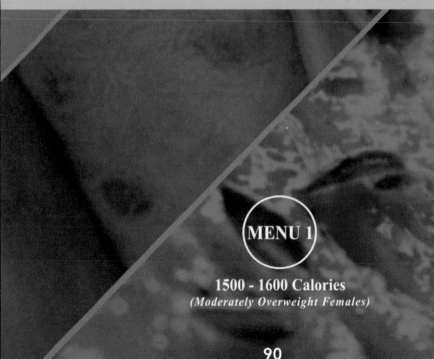

MENU 1

1500 - 1600 Calories
(Moderately Overweight Females)

3 DAY

Q
Dr. Quinn's
Dietary Recommendations
for Healthy Eating

☕ BREAKFAST

1 Vegetable & Cheese Omelet	
1 Egg, Scrambled	70 Calories, 0gm CHO, 5gm FAT, 6gm PRO
1 oz. Mozzarella Cheese	80 Calories, 0gm CHO, 6gm FAT, 7gm PRO
1/2 Cup Onions & Peppers, Sautéed	20 Calories, 3gm CHO, 0gm FAT, 1gm PRO
1/2 Cup Grits, Cooked	80 Calories, 15gm CHO, 2gm FAT, 2gm PRO
1/2 Cup Juice	60 Calories, 15gm CHO, 0gm FAT, 0gm PRO
1 Cup Coffee	2 Calories, 0gm CHO, 0gm FAT, 0gm PRO

Snack

1/2 English Muffin	60 Calories, 13gm CHO, 1gm FAT, 2gm PRO
1/2 Cup Nonfat Vanilla Yogurt	60 Calories, 10gm CHO, 0gm FAT, 6gm PRO
1 Cup Strawberries, Halved	60 Calories, 12gm CHO, 0gm FAT, 1gm PRO

🍴 LUNCH
Turkey Sandwich

2 oz. Turkey Breast	50 Calories, 1gm CHO, 1gm FAT, 9gm PRO
2 Pieces Whole Wheat Bread	160 Calories, 30gm CHO, 2gm FAT, 6gm PRO
1 Slice Tomato	5 Calories, 1gm CHO, 0gm FAT, 0gm PRO
1 oz. (1 Slice) Swiss Cheese	80 Calories, 0gm CHO, 6gm FAT, 6gm PRO
2 Slices Lettuce	5 Calories, 0gm CHO, 0gm FAT, 0gm PRO
1 Tbsp. Light Mayonnaise	35 Calories, 1gm CHO, 4gm FAT, 0gm PRO
1 tsp. Mustard	0 Calories, 0gm CHO, 0gm FAT, 0gm PRO
1 Bag Baked Chips (~12)	120 Calories, 22gm CHO, 3gm FAT, 2gm PRO

MENU 1

1500 - 1600 Calories
(Moderately Overweight Females)

3
DAY

Snack

2 Small Tangerine Oranges   60 Calories, 15gm CHO, 0gm FAT, 1gm PRO

DINNER

3 oz. Chicken Breast, Baked	105 Calories, 0gm CHO, 4gm FAT, 16gm PRO
12 Asparagus Spears, Broiled	40 Calories, 6gm CHO, 0gm FAT, 2gm PRO
2/3 Cup Brown Rice	160 Calories, 30gm CHO, 1gm FAT, 3gm PRO
2 Cups Mixed Green Salad	50 Calories, 10gm CHO, 0gm FAT, 2gm PRO
2 Tbsp. Light Italian Dressing	35 Calories, 3gm CHO, 3gm FAT, 0gm PRO

Snack

1 oz. Trail Mix   130 Calories, 13gm CHO, 8gm FAT, 4gm PRO

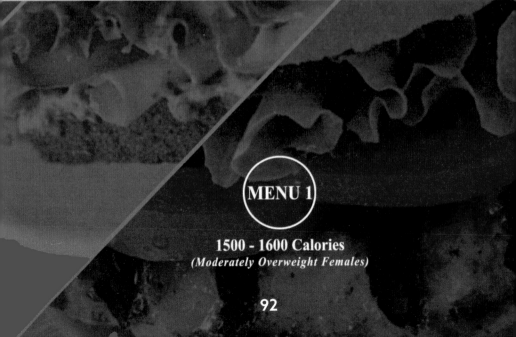

MENU 1

1500 - 1600 Calories
(Moderately Overweight Females)

Q
Dr. Quinn's
Dietary Recommendations for Healthy Eating

🍴 BREAKFAST

1 Piece Whole Wheat Toast	80 Calories, 15gm CHO, 1gm FAT, 3gm PRO
1 Vegetable Sausage	80 Calories, 3gm CHO, 3gm FAT, 10gm PRO
1 Tbsp. Grape Jelly	50 Calories, 13gm CHO, 0gm FAT, 0gm PRO
1 Cup Nonfat Flavored Yogurt	120 Calories, 19gm CHO, 0gm FAT, 12gm PRO

Snack

1/4 Cup Sunflower Kernels, No Added Salt	160 Calories, 6gm CHO, 14gm FAT, 6gm PRO

🍴 LUNCH

1 Veggie Burger

1 Hamburger Bun	120 Calories, 23gm CHO, 2gm FAT, 3gm PRO
1 Vegetable Burger	130 Calories, 5gm CHO, 6gm FAT, 15gm PRO
2 Slices Lettuce	5 Calories, 0gm CHO, 0gm FAT, 0gm PRO
1 Slice Tomato	5 Calories, 1gm CHO, 0gm FAT, 0gm PRO
1 Tbsp. Light Mayonnaise	35 Calories, 1gm CHO, 4gm FAT, 0gm PRO
1 tsp. Mustard	0 Calories, 0gm CHO, 0gm FAT, 0gm PRO
1/2 Cup Grapes	60 Calories, 15gm CHO, 0gm FAT, 1gm PRO

MENU 1

1500 - 1600 Calories
(Moderately Overweight Females)

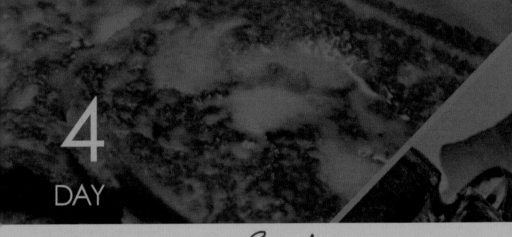

4
DAY

Snack

2 Tbsp. Hummus	70 Calories, 4gm CHO, 5gm FAT, 2gm PRO
1 Cup Carrot, Cucumber or Celery Sticks	25 Calories, 5gm CHO, 0gm FAT, 2gm PRO

🍴DINNER
1 Black Bean Taco*

1 Whole Wheat Tortilla Wrap	130 Calories, 22gm CHO, 3gm FAT, 3gm PR
¼ Cup Black Beans	50 Calories, 9gm CHO, 0gm FAT, 3gm PRO
¼ Cup Corn	30 Calories, 6gm CHO, 1gm FAT, 1gm PRO
¼ Cup Onions and Peppers, Roasted	10 Calories, 2gm CHO, 0gm FAT, 0gm PRO
1 oz. Mozzarella Cheese	80 Calories, 0gm CHO, 6gm FAT, 7gm PRO
2 Tbsp. Salsa	10 Calories, 3gm CHO, 0gm FAT, 0gm PRO
2 Cups Mixed Green Salad	50 Calories, 10gm CHO, 0gm FAT, 2gm PRO
2 Tbsp. Light Italian Dressing	35 Calories, 3gm CHO, 3gm FAT, 0gm PRO

Try Topping with Fresh, Chopped Cilantro or Lime Juice

Snack

1/2 Cup Cottage Cheese, Low Fat	90 Calories, 5gm CHO, 3gm FAT, 13gm PRO
1/2 Cup Fruit	60 Calories, 15gm CHO, 0gm FAT, 1gm PRO

MENU 1

1500 - 1600 Calories
(Moderately Overweight Females)

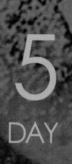

5
DAY

Q
Dr. Quinn's
Dietary Recommendations
for Healthy Eating

🍴 BREAKFAST

1 Pancake (4" Diameter)	80 Calories, 11gm CHO, 3gm FAT, 3gm PRO
1 Egg, Scrambled	70 Calories, 0gm CHO, 5gm FAT, 6gm PRO
1/2 Banana	45 Calories, 12gm CHO, 0gm FAT, 0gm PRO
1 Cup Skim Milk	80 Calories, 12gm CHO, 0gm FAT, 8gm PRO
2 Tbsp. Light Syrup	50 Calories, 13gm CHO, 0gm FAT, 0gm PRO

Snack

1 Cup Nonfat Flavored Yogurt	120 Calories, 19gm CHO, 0gm FAT, 12gm PRO

🍴 LUNCH

1 Chicken Salad Sandwich

1/2 Cup Chicken Salad	250 Calories, 8gm CHO, 16gm FAT, 17gm PRO
2 Pieces of Whole Wheat Bread	160 Calories, 30gm CHO, 2gm FAT, 6gm PRO
2 Slices Lettuce	5 Calories, 0gm CHO, 0gm FAT, 0gm PRO
1 Slice Tomato	5 Calories, 1gm CHO, 0gm FAT, 0gm PRO
4 to 6 Pita Crackers	90 Calories, 9gm CHO, 5gm FAT, 1gm PRO
2 Tbsp. Hummus	70 Calories, 4gm CHO, 5gm FAT, 2gm PRO

MENU 1

1500 - 1600 Calories
(Moderately Overweight Females)

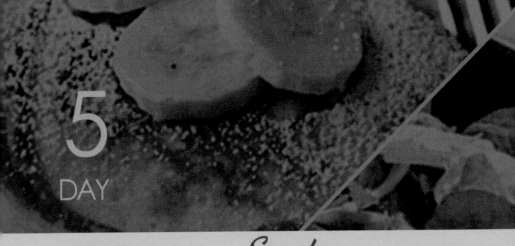

5
DAY

Snack

4 to 6 Crackers	90 Calories, 9gm CHO, 5gm FAT, 1gm PRO
2 oz. Tuna (Packed in Water)	50 Calories, 0gm CHO, 1gm FAT, 11gm PRO

DINNER
Spaghetti With Meat Sauce

1/3 Cup Spaghetti	80 Calories, 15gm CHO, 0gm FAT, 3gm PRO
1 oz. (2 Tbsp.) Ground Beef, Lean	60 Calories, 0gm CHO, 3gm FAT, 8gm PRO
1/3 Cup Marinara Sauce	50 Calories, 9gm CHO, 1gm FAT, 1gm PRO
1/2 Cup Green Beans	20 Calories, 4gm CHO, 0gm FAT, 1gm PRO
2 Cups Tossed Green Salad	50 Calories, 10gm CHO, 0gm FAT, 2gm PRO
2 Tbsp. Light Italian Dressing	35 Calories, 3gm CHO, 3gm FAT, 0gm PRO

Snack

1 Medium Apple	80 Calories, 22gm CHO, 0gm FAT, 0gm PRO

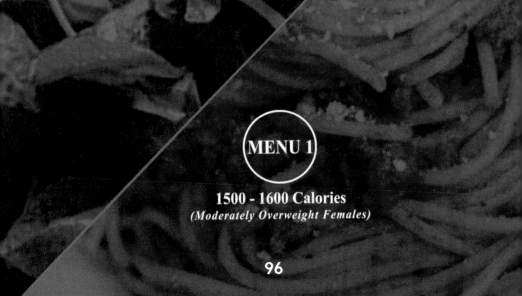

MENU 1

1500 - 1600 Calories
(Moderately Overweight Females)

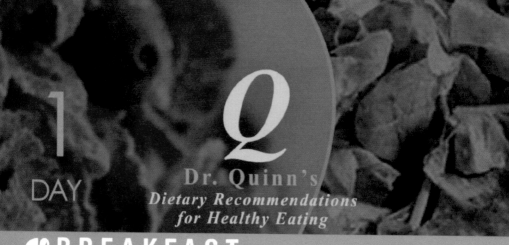

1 DAY

Q
Dr. Quinn's
*Dietary Recommendations
for Healthy Eating*

🍴 BREAKFAST

¾ Cup Cereal, Un-Sweetened	100 Calories, 22gm CHO, 1gm FAT, 2gm PRO
2 Hardboiled Eggs	140 Calories, 0gm CHO, 10gm FAT, 12gm PRO
1 Small Orange	60 Calories, 15gm CHO, 0gm FAT, 1gm PRO
1 Cup Skim Milk	80 Calories, 12gm CHO, 0gm FAT, 8gm PRO
1 Cup Coffee	2 Calories, 0gm CHO, 0gm FAT, 0gm PRO

Snack

1 Small Banana	90 Calories, 23gm CHO, 0gm FAT, 1gm PRO
2 Tbsp. Peanut Butter	190 Calories, 8gm CHO, 16gm FAT, 7gm PRO

🍴 LUNCH

2 Cups Low Sodium Tomato Soup	150 Calories, 32gm CHO, 2gm FAT, 4gm PRO
4 to 6 Crackers	90 Calories, 9gm CHO, 5gm FAT, 1gm PRO
2 Cups Mixed Green Salad	50 Calories, 10gm CHO, 0gm FAT, 2gm PRO
2 Tbsp. Light Ranch Dressing	80 Calories, 3gm CHO, 7gm FAT, 1gm PRO

Snack

1 oz. Mixed Nuts	170 Calories, 6gm CHO, 15gm FAT, 6gm PRO

MENU 2

1800 - 1900 Calories
(Very Overweight Females and/or Moderately Overweight Males)

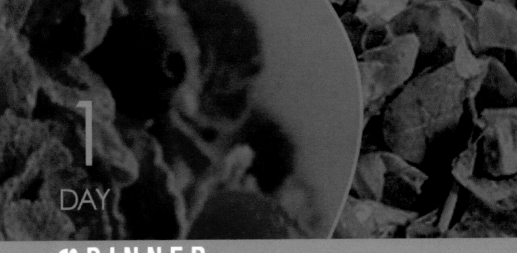

1 DAY

🍴 DINNER

3 oz. Pork Loin, Baked	165 Calories, 0gm CHO, 2gm FAT, 17gm PRO
1 Cup (~10) Brussels Sprouts, (Baked)	90 Calories, 15gm CHO, 0gm FAT, 6gm PRO
1 Cup Black-Eyed Peas	180 Calories, 30gm CHO, 2gm FAT, 10gm PRO
1 Small Dinner Roll	80 Calories, 15gm CHO, 1gm FAT, 3gm PRO

Snack

1 Cup Nonfat Flavored Yogurt	120 Calories, 19gm CHO, 0gm FAT, 12gm PRO
1/2 Cup Strawberries, Sliced	30 Calories, 7gm CHO, 0gm FAT, 1gm PRO

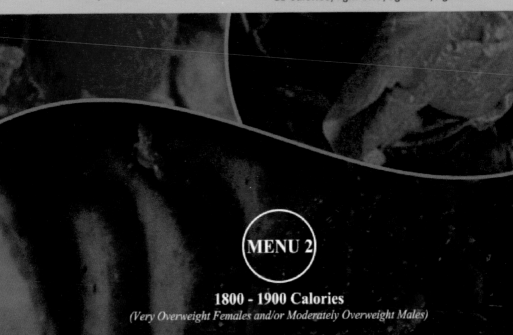

MENU 2

1800 - 1900 Calories
(Very Overweight Females and/or Moderately Overweight Males)

2
DAY

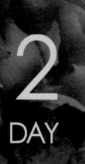

Q
Dr. Quinn's
Dietary Recommendations
for Healthy Eating

🍴BREAKFAST

1 Cup Oatmeal, Cooked	150 Calories, 27gm CHO, 2gm FAT, 5gm PRO
1/2 Cup Fresh or Frozen Blueberries	42 Calories, 11gm CHO, 0gm FAT, 1gm PRO
1 Vegetable Breakfast Sausage	80 Calories, 3gm CHO, 3gm FAT, 10gm PRO
1 Cup Skim Milk	80 Calories, 12gm CHO, 0gm FAT, 8gm PRO
1 Cup Coffee	2 Calories, 0gm CHO, 0gm FAT, 0gm PRO

Snack

4 to 6 Crackers	90 Calories, 9gm CHO, 5gm FAT, 1gm PRO
1 Mozzarella String Cheese	80 Calories, 0gm CHO, 6gm FAT, 7gm PRO

🍴LUNCH

1 Chicken Wrap With Fresh Vegetables

1 Whole Wheat Tortilla Wrap	130 Calories, 22gm CHO, 3gm FAT, 3gm PRO
3 oz. Chicken Breast, Chopped	105 Calories, 0gm CHO, 4gm FAT, 16gm PRO
1/2 Cup Mixed Vegetables, Roasted	25 Calories, 5gm CHO, 0gm FAT, 1gm PRO
2 Tbsp. Light Ranch Dressing	80 Calories, 3gm CHO, 7gm FAT, 1gm PRO
1 Small Bag of Pretzels (17)	110 Calories, 23gm CHO, 1gm FAT, 3gm PRO
2 Tbsp. Hummus	70 Calories, 4gm CHO, 5gm FAT, 2gm PRO

Snack

1 Cup Nonfat Flavored Yogurt	120 Calories, 19gm CHO, 0gm FAT, 12gm PRO
2 Tbsp. Granola	60 Calories, 10gm CHO, 2gm FAT, 1gm PRO

MENU 2

1800 - 1900 Calories
(Very Overweight Females and/or Moderately Overweight Males)

2
DAY

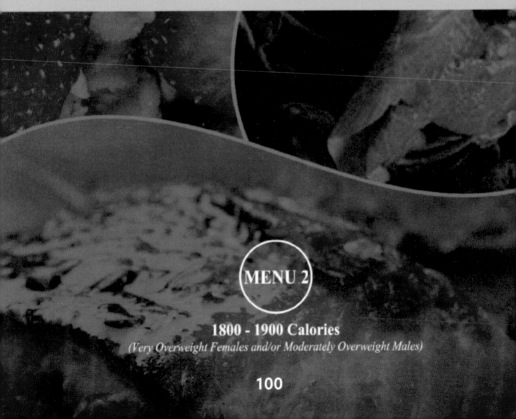

🍴DINNER

3 oz. Salmon, Baked	130 Calories, 0gm CHO, 5gm FAT, 21gm PRO
1 Cup Red Potato Wedges, Baked	160 Calories, 30gm CHO, 0gm FAT, 6gm PRO
1 Small Dinner Roll	80 Calories, 15gm CHO, 1gm FAT, 3gm PRO
2 Cups Mixed Green Salad	50 Calories, 10gm CHO, 0gm FAT, 2gm PRO
2 Tbsp. Light Italian Dressing	35 Calories, 3gm CHO, 3gm FAT, 0gm PRO

Snack

1 Medium Apple	80 Calories, 22gm CHO, 0gm FAT, 0gm PRO
1 Tbsp. Peanut Butter	95 Calories, 4gm CHO, 8gm FAT, 4gm PRO

MENU 2

1800 - 1900 Calories
(Very Overweight Females and/or Moderately Overweight Males)

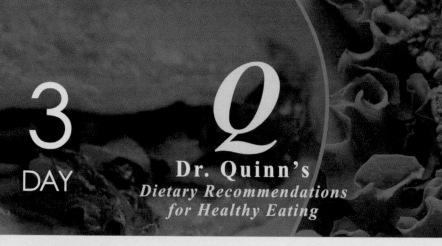

3 DAY

Q
Dr. Quinn's
Dietary Recommendations for Healthy Eating

🍴BREAKFAST
1 Vegetable & Cheese Omelet

1 Egg, Scrambled	70 Calories, 0gm CHO, 5gm FAT, 6gm PRO
1 oz. Mozzarella Cheese	80 Calories, 0gm CHO, 6gm FAT, 7gm PRO
1/2 Cup Onions & Peppers, Sautéed	20 Calories, 3gm CHO, 0gm FAT, 1gm PRO
1/2 Cup Grits, Cooked	80 Calories, 15gm CHO, 2gm FAT, 2gm PRO
1/2 Cup Juice	60 Calories, 15gm CHO, 0gm FAT, 0gm PRO
1 Cup Skim Milk	80 Calories, 12gm CHO, 0gm FAT 8gm PRO
1 Cup Coffee	2 Calories, 0gm CHO, 0gm FAT, 0gm PRO

Snack

1/2 English Muffin	60 Calories, 13gm CHO, 1gm FAT, 2gm PRO
1/2 Cup Nonfat Vanilla Yogurt	60 Calories, 10gm CHO, 0gm FAT, 6gm PRO
1 Cup Strawberries, Halved	60 Calories, 12gm CHO, 0gm FAT, 1gm PRO

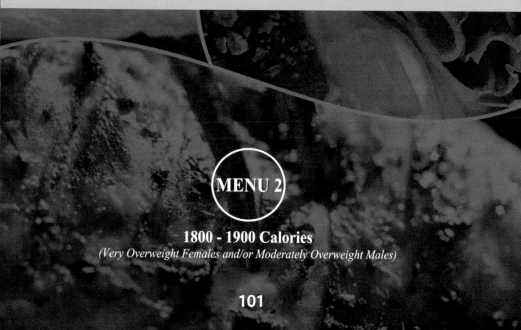

MENU 2

1800 - 1900 Calories
(Very Overweight Females and/or Moderately Overweight Males)

3

DAY

🍴 LUNCH

Turkey Sandwich

2 oz. Turkey Breast	50 Calories, 1gm CHO, 1gm FAT, 9gm PRO
2 Pieces Whole Wheat Bread	160 Calories, 30gm CHO, 2gm FAT, 6gm PRO
1 Slice Tomato	5 Calories, 1gm CHO, 0gm FAT, 0gm PRO
1 oz. (1 Slice) Swiss Cheese	80 Calories, 0gm CHO, 6gm FAT, 6gm PRO
2 Slices Lettuce	5 Calories, 0gm CHO, 0gm FAT, 0gm PRO
1 Tbsp. Light Mayonnaise	35 Calories, 1gm CHO, 4gm FAT, 0gm PRO
1 tsp. Mustard	0 Calories, 0gm CHO, 0gm FAT, 0gm PRO
1 Bag Baked chips (~12)	120 Calories, 22gm CHO, 3gm FAT, 2gm PRO
2 Tbsp. Hummus	70 Calories, 4gm CHO, 5gm FAT, 2gm PRO

Snack

3 Small Tangerine Oranges	90 Calories, 23gm CHO, 0gm FAT, 1gm PRO

🍴 DINNER

3 oz. Chicken Breast, Baked	105 Calories, 0gm CHO, 4gm FAT, 16gm PRO
12 Asparagus Spears, Broiled	40 Calories, 6gm CHO, 0gm FAT, 2gm PRO
2/3 Cup Brown Rice	160 Calories, 30gm CHO, 1gm FAT, 3gm PRO
2 Cups Mixed Green Salad	50 Calories, 10gm CHO, 0gm FAT, 2gm PRO
2 Tbsp. Light Italian Dressing	35 Calories, 3gm CHO, 3gm FAT, 0gm PRO
1 Small Dinner Roll	80 Calories, 15gm CHO, 1gm FAT, 3gm PRO
1 tsp. Margarine	30 Calories, 0gm CHO, 4gm FAT, 0gm PRO

Snack

1 oz. Trail Mix	130 Calories, 13gm CHO, 8gm FAT, 4gm PRO

MENU 2

1800 - 1900 Calories
(Very Overweight Females and/or Moderately Overweight Males)

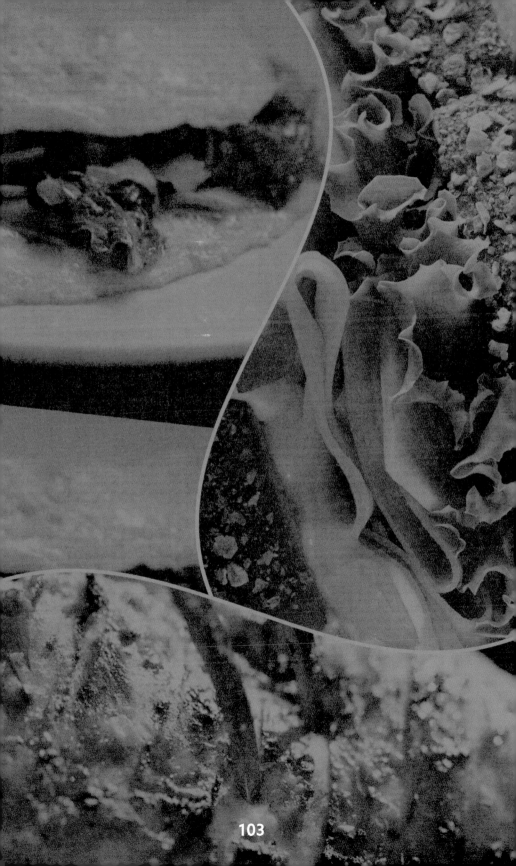

4 DAY

Q Dr. Quinn's
Dietary Recommendations for Healthy Eating

🍴BREAKFAST

1 Piece Whole Wheat Toast	80 Calories, 15gm CHO, 1gm FAT, 3gm PRO
1 Vegetable Sausage	80 Calories, 3gm CHO, 3gm FAT, 10gm PRO
1 Tbsp. Grape Jelly	50 Calories, 13gm CHO, 0gm FAT, 0gm PRO
1 Cup Skim Milk	80 Calories, 12gm CHO, 0gm FAT, 8gm PRO

Snack

1/4 Cup Sunflower Kernels, No Added Salt	160 Calories, 6gm CHO, 14gm FAT, 6gm PRO
1 Small Box of Raisins	130 Calories, 34gm CHO, 0gm FAT, 1gm PRO

🍴LUNCH

1 Veggie Burger

1 Hamburger Bun	120 Calories, 23gm CHO, 2gm FAT, 3gm PRO
1 Vegetable Burger	130 Calories, 5gm CHO, 6gm FAT, 15gm PRO
2 Slices Lettuce	5 Calories, 0gm CHO, 0gm FAT, 0gm PRO
1 Slice Tomato	5 Calories, 1gm CHO, 0gm FAT, 0gm PRO
1 Tbsp. Light Mayonnaise	35 Calories, 1gm CHO, 4gm FAT, 0gm PRO
1 tsp. Mustard	0 Calories, 0gm CHO, 0gm FAT, 0gm PRO
1/2 Cup Cole Slaw	150 Calories, 15gm CHO, 10gm FAT, 1gm PRO
1/2 Cup Grapes	60 Calories, 15gm CHO, 0gm FAT, 1gm PRO

MENU 2

1800 - 1900 Calories
(Very Overweight Females and/or Moderately Overweight Males)

104

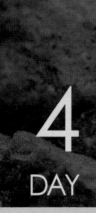

4
DAY

Snack

2 Tbsp. Hummus	70 Calories, 4gm CHO, 5gm FAT, 2gm PRO
1 Cup Carrot, Cucumber, or Celery Sticks	25 Calories, 5gm CHO, 0gm FAT, 2gm PRO

🍴DINNER
1 Black Bean Taco*

1 Whole Wheat Tortilla Wrap	130 Calories, 22gm CHO, 3gm FAT, 3gm PRO
1/4 Cup Black Beans	50 Calories, 9gm CHO, 0gm FAT, 3gm PRO
1/4 Cup Corn	30 Calories, 6gm CHO, 1gm FAT, 1gm PRO
1/4 Cup Onions And Peppers, Roasted	10 Calories, 2gm CHO, 0gm FAT, 0gm PRO
1 oz. Mozzarella Cheese	80 Calories, 0gm CHO, 6gm FAT, 7gm PRO
2 Tbsp. Salsa	10 Calories, 3gm CHO, 0gm FAT, 0gm PRO
2 Cups Tossed Green Salad	50 Calories, 10gm CHO, 0gm FAT, 2gm PRO
2 Tbsp. Light Ranch Dressing	80 Calories, 3gm CHO, 7gm FAT, 1gm PRO

 Try Topping with Fresh, Chopped Cilantro or Lime Juice

Snack

1 Cup Cottage Cheese, Low Fat	180 Calories, 10gm CHO, 6gm FAT, 26gm PRO
1/2 Cup Fruit	60 Calories, 15gm CHO, 0gm FAT, 1gm PRO

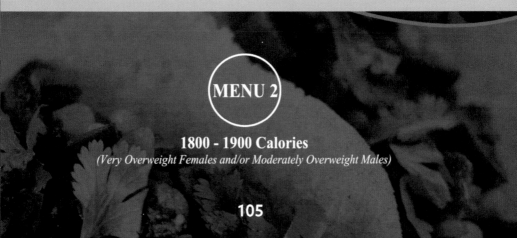

MENU 2

1800 - 1900 Calories
(Very Overweight Females and/or Moderately Overweight Males)

Q
Dr. Quinn's
Dietary Recommendations
for Healthy Eating

BREAKFAST

2 Pancakes (4" diameter)	160 Calories, 22gm CHO, 6gm FAT, 6gm PRO
1 Egg, Scrambled	70 Calories, 0gm CHO, 5gm FAT, 6gm PRO
1 Cup Skim Milk	80 Calories, 12gm CHO, 0gm FAT, 8gm PRO
2 Tbsp. Light Syrup	50 Calories, 13gm CHO, 0gm FAT, 0gm PRO

Snack

1 Cup Nonfat Flavored Yogurt	120 Calories, 19gm CHO, 0gm FAT, 12gm PRO
1/2 Banana	45 Calories, 12gm CHO, 0gm FAT, 0gm PRO

LUNCH

1 Chicken Salad Sandwich

1/2 Cup Chicken Salad	250 Calories, 8gm CHO, 16gm FAT, 17gm PRO
2 Pieces Whole Wheat Bread	160 Calories, 30gm CHO, 2gm FAT, 6gm PRO
2 Slices Lettuce	5 Calories, 0gm CHO, 0gm FAT, 0gm PRO
1 Slice Tomato	5 Calories, 1gm CHO, 0gm FAT, 0gm PRO
4 to 6 Pita Crackers	90 Calories, 9gm CHO, 5gm FAT, 1gm PRO

MENU 2

1800 - 1900 Calories
(Very Overweight Females and/or Moderately Overweight Males)

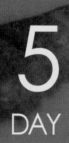

5
DAY

Snack

2 oz. Tuna (Packed in Water)	50 Calories, 0gm CHO, 1gm FAT, 11gm PRO
4 to 6 Crackers	90 Calories, 9gm CHO, 5gm FAT, 1gm PRO

🍴DINNER
Spaghetti with Meat Sauce

2/3 Cup Spaghetti	160 Calories, 30gm CHO, 1gm FAT, 6gm PRO
2 oz. (1/4 Cup) Ground Beef, Lean	120 Calories, 0gm CHO, 6gm FAT, 16gm PRO
1/2 Cup Marinara Sauce	70 Calories, 13gm CHO, 2gm FAT, 2gm PRO
1/2 Cup Green Beans	20 Calories, 4gm CHO, 0gm FAT, 1gm PRO
2 Cups Mixed Green Salad	50 Calories, 10gm CHO, 0gm FAT, 2gm PRO
2 Tbsp. Light Italian Dressing	35 Calories, 3gm CHO, 3gm FAT, 0gm PRO

Snack

1 Medium Apple	80 Calories, 22gm CHO, 0gm FAT, 0gm PRO
1 Tbsp. Peanut Butter	95 Calories, 4gm CHO, 8gm FAT, 4gm PRO

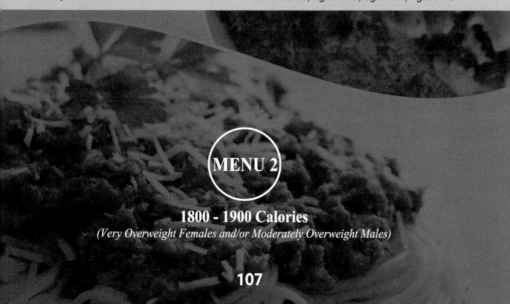

MENU 2

1800 - 1900 Calories

(Very Overweight Females and/or Moderately Overweight Males)

Q
Dr. Quinn's
Dietary Recommendations
for Healthy Eating

BREAKFAST

3/4 Cup Cereal, Un-Sweetened	100 Calories, 22gm CHO, 1gm FAT, 2gm PRO
2 Hardboiled Eggs	140 Calories, 0gm CHO, 10gm FAT, 12gm PRO
1 Small Orange	60 Calories, 15gm CHO, 0gm FAT, 1gm PRO
1 Cup Skim Milk	80 Calories, 12gm CHO, 0gm FAT, 8gm PRO
1 Cup Coffee	2 Calories, 0gm CHO, 0gm FAT, 0gm PRO

Snack

1 Small Banana	90 Calories, 23gm CHO, 0gm FAT, 1gm PRO
2 Tbsp. Peanut Butter	190 Calories, 8gm CHO, 16gm FAT, 7gm PRO

LUNCH

2 Cups Low Sodium Tomato Soup	150 Calories, 32gm CHO, 2gm FAT, 4gm PRO
4 to 6 Crackers	90 Calories, 9gm CHO, 5gm FAT, 1gm PRO
2 Cups Mixed Green Salad	50 Calories, 10gm CHO, 0gm FAT, 2gm PRO
2 Tbsp. Light Ranch Dressing	80 Calories, 3gm CHO, 7gm FAT, 1gm PRO

Snack

1 oz. Mixed Nuts	170 Calories, 6gm CHO, 15gm FAT, 6gm PRO
1 Small Box of Raisins	130 Calories, 34gm CHO, 0gm FAT, 1gm PRO

MENU 3

2,000 - 2,200 Calories
(Very Overweight Males)

1 DAY

(Î)DINNER

3 oz. Pork Loin, Baked	165 Calories, 0gm CHO, 2gm FAT, 17gm PRO
1 Cup (10) Brussels Sprouts, Baked	90 Calories, 15gm CHO, 0gm FAT, 6gm PRO
1 Cup Black-Eyed Peas	180 Calories, 30gm CHO, 2gm FAT, 10gm PRO
1 Small Dinner Roll	80 Calories, 15gm CHO, 1gm FAT, 3gm PRO
1 tsp. Margarine	30 Calories, 0gm CHO, 4gm FAT, 0gm PRO

Snack

1 Cup Nonfat Vanilla Yogurt	120 Calories, 19gm CHO, 0gm FAT, 12gm PRO
1/4 Cup of Granola	120 Calories, 19gm CHO, 4gm FAT, 3gm PRO

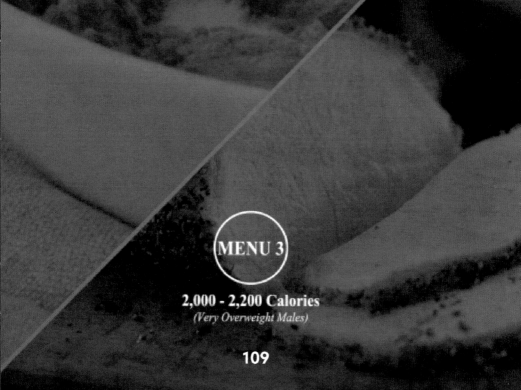

MENU 3

2,000 - 2,200 Calories
(Very Overweight Males)

2 DAY

Q

Dr. Quinn's
Dietary Recommendations
for Healthy Eating

🍴BREAKFAST

1 Cup Oatmeal, Cooked	150 Calories, 27gm CHO, 2gm FAT, 5gm PRO
1/2 Cup Fresh or Frozen Blueberries	42 Calories, 11gm CHO, 0gm FAT, 1gm PRO
1 Vegetable Breakfast Sausage	80 Calories, 3gm CHO, 3gm FAT, 10gm PRO
1 Cup Skim Milk	80 Calories, 12gm CHO, 0gm FAT, 8gm PRO
1/2 Cup of Juice	60 Calories, 15gm CHO, 0gm FAT, 0gm PRO

Snack

4 to 6 Crackers	90 Calories, 9gm CHO, 5gm FAT, 1gm PRO
1 Mozzarella String Cheese	80 Calories, 0gm CHO, 6gm FAT, 7gm PRO

🍴LUNCH

1 Chicken Wrap With Fresh Vegetables

1 Whole Wheat Tortilla Wrap	130 Calories, 22gm CHO, 3gm FAT, 3gm PRO
3 oz. Chicken Breast, Chopped	105 Calories, 0gm CHO, 4gm FAT, 16gm PRO
1/2 Cup Mixed Vegetables, Roasted	25 Calories, 5gm CHO, 0gm FAT, 1gm PRO
2 Tbsp. Light Ranch Dressing	80 Calories, 3gm CHO, 7gm FAT, 1gm PRO
1 Small Bag of Pretzels (17)	110 Calories, 23gm CHO, 1gm FAT, 3gm PRO
2 Tbsp. Hummus	70 Calories, 4gm CHO, 5gm FAT, 2gm PRO

Snack

1 Cup Nonfat Flavored Yogurt	120 Calories, 19gm CHO, 0gm FAT, 12gm PRO
1/4 Cup Granola	120 Calories, 19gm CHO, 4gm FAT, 3gm PRO

MENU 3

2,000 - 2,200 Calories
(Very Overweight Males)

2
DAY

⏾DINNER

4 oz. Salmon, Baked	175 Calories, 0gm CHO, 6gm FAT, 28gm PRO
1 Cup Red Potato Wedges, Baked	160 Calories, 30gm CHO, 0gm FAT, 6gm PRO
2 Cups Mixed Green Salad	50 Calories, 10gm CHO, 0gm FAT, 2gm PRO
2 Tbsp. Light Italian Dressing	35 Calories, 3gm CHO, 3gm FAT, 0gm PRO
1 Small Dinner Roll	80 Calories, 15gm CHO, 1gm FAT, 3gm PRO

Snack

1 Medium Apple	80 Calories, 22gm CHO, 0gm FAT, 0gm PRO
2 Tbsp. Peanut Butter	190 Calories, 8gm CHO, 16gm FAT, 7gm PRO

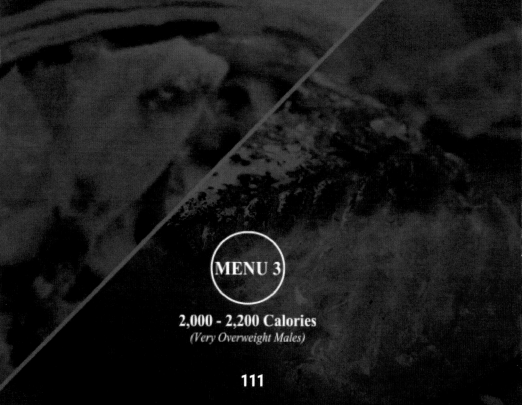

MENU 3

2,000 - 2,200 Calories
(Very Overweight Males)

3 DAY

Q
Dr. Quinn's
Dietary Recommendations
for Healthy Eating

BREAKFAST
1 Vegetable & Cheese Omelet

1 Egg, Scrambled	70 Calories, 0gm CHO, 5gm FAT, 6gm PRO
1 oz. Mozzarella Cheese	80 Calories, 0gm CHO, 6gm FAT, 7gm PRO
1/2 Cup Onions & Peppers, Sautéed	20 Calories, 3gm CHO, 0gm FAT, 1gm PRO
1/2 Cup Grits, Cooked	80 Calories, 15gm CHO, 2gm FAT, 2gm PRO
1/2 Cup Juice	60 Calories, 15gm CHO, 0gm FAT, 0gm PRO
1 Cup Skim Milk	80 Calories, 12gm CHO, 0gm FAT, 8gm PRO
1 Cup Coffee	2 Calories, 0gm CHO, 0gm FAT, 0gm PRO

Snack

1/2 English Muffin	60 Calories, 13gm CHO, 1gm FAT, 2gm PRO
1/2 Cup Nonfat Vanilla Yogurt	60 Calories, 10gm CHO, 0gm FAT, 6gm PRO
1 Cup Strawberries, Halved	60 Calories, 12gm CHO, 0gm FAT, 1gm PRO
1 Tbsp. Almonds, Sliced	85 Calories, 3gm CHO, 3gm FAT, 3gm PRO

MENU 3

2,000 - 2,200 Calories
(Very Overweight Males)

3
DAY

((| LUNCH

Turkey Sandwich

2 oz. Turkey Breast	50 Calories, 1gm CHO, 1gm FAT, 9gm PRO
2 Pieces Whole Wheat Bread	160 Calories, 30gm CHO, 2gm FAT, 6gm PRO
1 Slice Tomato	5 Calories, 1gm CHO, 0gm FAT, 0gm PRO
1 oz. (1 slice) Swiss Cheese	80 Calories, 0gm CHO, 6gm FAT, 6gm PRO
2 slices Lettuce	5 Calories, 0gm CHO, 0gm FAT, 0gm PRO
1 Tbsp. Light Mayonnaise	35 Calories, 1gm CHO, 4gm FAT, 0gm PRO
1 tsp. Mustard	0 Calories, 0gm CHO, 0gm FAT, 0gm PRO
1 Bag of Baked Chips (~12)	120 Calories, 22gm CHO, 3gm FAT, 2gm PRO
2 Tbsp. Hummus	70 Calories, 4gm CHO, 5gm FAT, 2gm PRO
1 Cup Carrot, Cucumber, Or Celery Stalks	25 Calories, 5gm CHO, 0gm FAT, 2gm PRO

Snack

2 oz. Trail Mix	260 Calories, 26gm CHO, 16gm FAT, 8gm PRO

MENU 3

2,000 - 2,200 Calories
(Very Overweight Males)

3
DAY

❙❙DINNER

3 oz. Chicken Breast, Baked	105 Calories, 0gm CHO, 4gm FAT, 16gm PRO
12 Asparagus Spears, Broiled	40 Calories, 6gm CHO, 0gm FAT, 2gm PRO
2/3 Cup Brown Rice	160 Calories, 30gm CHO, 1gm FAT, 3gm PRO
2 Cups Mixed Green Salad	50 Calories, 10gm CHO, 0gm FAT, 2gm PRO
2 Tbsp. Light Italian Dressing	35 Calories, 3gm CHO, 3gm FAT, 0gm PRO
1 Small Dinner Roll	80 Calories, 15gm CHO, 1gm FAT, 3gm PRO
1 tsp. Margarine	30 Calories, 0gm CHO, 4gm FAT, 0gm PRO

Snack

3 Small Tangerine Oranges	90 Calories, 23gm CHO, 0gm FAT, 1gm PRO

MENU 3

2,000 - 2,200 Calories
(Very Overweight Males)

4
DAY

Q
Dr. Quinn's
Dietary Recommendations
for Healthy Eating

🍴 B R E A K F A S T

1 Piece Whole Wheat Toast	80 Calories, 15gm CHO, 1gm FAT, 3gm PRO
1 Vegetable Sausage	80 Calories, 3gm CHO, 3gm FAT, 10gm PRO
1/2 Cup Grits, Cooked	80 Calories, 15gm CHO, 2gm FAT, 2gm PRO
1/2 Cup Skim Milk	40 Calories, 6gm CHO, 0gm FAT, 4gm PRO
1 Tbsp. Grape Jelly	50 Calories, 13gm CHO, 0gm FAT, 0gm PRO

Snack

1/4 Cup Sunflower Kernels, No Added Salt	160 Calories, 6gm CHO, 14gm FAT, 6gm PRO
1 Small Box of Raisins	130 Calories, 34gm CHO, 0gm FAT, 1gm PRO

🍴 L U N C H
1 Veggie Burger

1 Hamburger Bun	120 Calories, 23gm CHO, 2gm FAT, 3gm PRO
1 Vegetable Burger	130 Calories, 5gm CHO, 6gm FAT, 15gm PRO
1 oz. American Cheese (1 Slice)	70 Calories, 2gm CHO, 5gm FAT, 4gm PRO
2 Slices Lettuce	5 Calories, 0gm CHO, 0gm FAT, 0gm PRO
1 Slice Tomato	5 Calories, 1gm CHO, 0gm FAT, 0gm PRO
1 Tbsp. Light Mayonnaise	35 Calories, 1gm CHO, 4gm FAT, 0gm PRO
1 tsp. Mustard	0 Calories, 0gm CHO, 0gm FAT, 0gm PRO
1/2 Cup Cole Slaw	150 Calories, 15gm CHO, 10gm FAT, 1gm PRO
1/2 Cup Grapes	60 Calories, 15gm CHO, 0gm FAT, 1gm PRO

MENU 3

2,000 - 2,200 Calories
(Very Overweight Males)

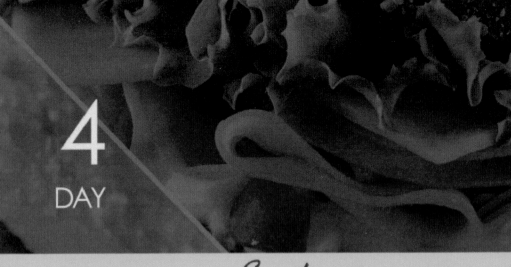

4
DAY

Snack

2 Tbsp. Hummus	70 Calories, 4gm CHO, 5gm FAT, 2gm PRO
1 Cup Carrot, Cucumber, or Celery Sticks	25 Calories, 5gm CHO, 0gm FAT, 2gm PRO

DINNER
1 Black Bean Taco*

1 Whole Wheat Tortilla Wrap	130 Calories, 22gm CHO, 3gm FAT, 3gm PRO
1/4 Cup Black Beans	50 Calories, 9gm CHO, 0gm FAT, 3gm PRO
1/4 Cup Corn	30 Calories, 6gm CHO, 1gm FAT, 1gm PRO
1/4 Cup Onions And Peppers, Roasted	10 Calories, 2gm CHO, 0gm FAT, 0gm PRO
1 oz. Mozzarella Cheese	80 Calories, 0gm CHO, 6gm FAT, 7gm PRO
2 Tbsp. Salsa	10 Calories, 3gm CHO, 0gm FAT, 0gm PRO
1/3 Cup Brown Rice*	80 Calories, 15gm CHO, 1gm FAT, 1gm PRO
1 Cup Mixed Green Salad	25 Calories, 5gm CHO, 0gm FAT, 1gm PRO
1 Tbsp. Light Ranch Dressing	40 Calories, 2gm CHO, 3gm FAT, 0gm PRO

Try Topping with Fresh, Chopped Cilantro or Lime Juice

Snack

1 Cup Cottage Cheese, Low Fat	180 Calories, 10gm CHO, 6gm FAT, 26gm PRO
1/2 Cup Fruit	60 Calories, 15gm CHO, 0gm FAT, 1gm PRO

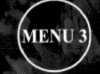

MENU 3

2,000 - 2,200 Calories
(Very Overweight Males)

5 DAY

Q

Dr. Quinn's
Dietary Recommendations for Healthy Eating

🍴 BREAKFAST

2 Pancakes (4" diameter)	160 Calories, 22gm CHO, 6gm FAT, 6gm PRO
1 Egg, Scrambled	70 Calories, 0gm CHO, 5gm FAT, 6gm PRO
1 Slice Bacon	40 Calories, 0gm CHO, 3gm FAT, 3gm PRO
1 Small Orange	60 Calories, 15gm CHO, 0gm FAT, 1gm PRO
1 Cup Skim Milk	80 Calories, 12gm CHO, 0gm FAT, 8gm PRO
2 Tbsp. Light Syrup	50 Calories, 13gm CHO, 0gm FAT, 0gm PRO

Snack

1 Cup Nonfat Flavored Yogurt	120 Calories, 19gm CHO, 0gm FAT, 12gm PRO
1/4 Cup Granola	120 Calories, 19gmCHO, 4gm FAT, 3gm PRO

🍴 LUNCH

1 Chicken Salad Sandwich

1/2 Cup Chicken Salad	250 Calories, 8gm CHO, 16gm FAT, 17gm PRO
2 Pieces Whole Wheat Bread	160 Calories, 30gm CHO, 2gm FAT, 6gm PRO
2 Slices Lettuce	5 Calories, 0gm CHO, 0gm FAT, 0gm PRO
1 Slice Tomato	5 Calories, 1gm CHO, 0gm FAT, 0gm PRO
4 to 6 Pita Crackers	90 Calories, 9gm CHO, 5gm FAT, 1gm PRO
2 Tbsp. Hummus	70 Calories, 4gm CHO, 5gm FAT, 2gm PRO

Snack

3 oz. Tuna (Packed in Water)	75 Calories, 0gm CHO, 2gm FAT, 17gm PRO
4 to 6 Crackers	90 Calories, 9gm CHO, 5gm FAT, 1gm PRO

MENU 3

2,000 - 2,200 Calories
(Very Overweight Males)

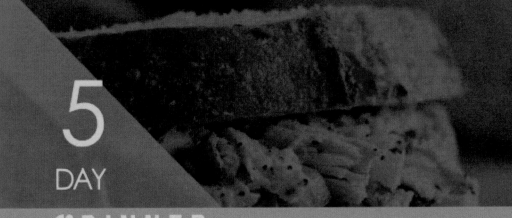

5
DAY

(I) D I N N E R
Spaghetti With Meat Sauce

2/3 Cup Spaghetti	160 Calories, 30gm CHO, 1gm FAT, 6gm PRO
2 oz. (1/4 cup) Ground Beef, Lean	120 Calories, 0gm CHO, 6gm FAT, 16gm PRO
1/2 Cup Marinara Sauce	70 Calories, 13gm CHO, 2gm FAT, 2gm PRO
1/2 Cup Green Beans	20 Calories, 4gm CHO, 0gm FAT, 1gm PRO
2 Cups Tossed Green Salad	50 Calories, 10gm CHO, 0gm FAT, 2gm PRO
2 Tbsp. Light Italian Dressing	35 Calories, 3gm CHO, 3gm FAT, 0gm PRO

Snack

1 Medium Apple	80 Calories, 22gm CHO, 0gm FAT, 0gm PRO
1 Tbsp. Peanut Butter	95 Calories, 4gm CHO, 8gm FAT, 4gm PRO

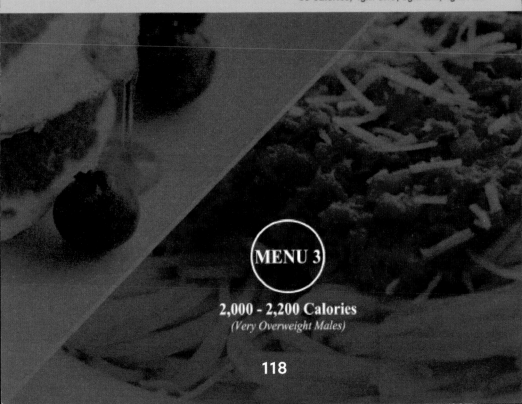

MENU 3

2,000 - 2,200 Calories
(Very Overweight Males)

THE PEOPLE'S DOCTOR
CONNECT WITH US ON
SOCIAL MEDIA

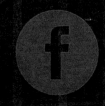

Dr. Timothy Quinn

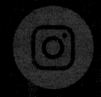

@AskDrQuinn

Timothy Quinn

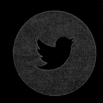

@AskDrQuinn

CREDITS

AUTHOR
TIMOTHY QUINN, M.D.
WWW.ASKDRQUINN.COM

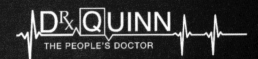

@AskDrQuinn   Timothy Quinn   Dr. Timothy Quinn   @AskDrQuinn

---

GRAPHICS | ILLUSTRATIONS |
BOOK DESIGN | CONTENT DEVELOPMENT EDITING
SONNIE DESIGN
Owner - Denise Terry
WWW.SONNIEDESIGN.COM | INFO@SONNIEDESIGN.COM

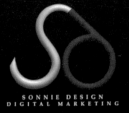

Sonnie Design   @SonnieDesign

GYM WORKOUT & HOME WORKOUT
Martin Fitness Solutions, LLC
Owner - James Martin
MS - ACSM Certified Exercise Physiologist &
NASM Certified Personal Trainer
JAMART30@HOTMAIL.COM | 662.242.0520

ENDORSEMENTS

Dr. Timothy Quinn is one of McComb, Mississippi's finest native sons. I am proud of Dr. Quinn and his many accomplishments. I'm especially proud of his successes in advocating the need for all people to live healthier lifestyles. *Mayor Whitney Rawlings, City of McComb*

Dr. Quinn is a professional with the flair for making things simple.

We turn to him as a medical expert because we know we can trust him! *Ben Hart, WAPT News Director, Jackson, MS*

Dr. Quinn has been an outstanding asset to our radio programming by providing the "Hip-Hop Medical Minute" to our young urban listening audience, who receive weekly much-needed health information. *Gregory K. McCoy, Operations Manager, WRBJ 97.7 FM Radio*

As a family-medicine physician, Dr. Timothy Quinn goes the extra mile to empower patients with the tools they need to achieve ultimate wellness. Focused on prevention and leading by example, Dr. Quinn tirelessly works within his practice and in several leadership positions throughout the community to emphasize and emanate the importance of total health and how one can achieve it. Whether it's volunteering his time to screen patients after their Sunday worship service or organizing events for local parents to learn more about health issues impacting their children, Dr. Quinn is clearly dedicated to improving the overall health of the greater Jackson metropolitan area. **Jon-Paul Croom, CEO of Merit Health Central Hospital**

As a public-health professional of the Mississippi State Department Health, I understand there are multiple factors at different levels (the individual, the interpersonal level, the community, society) that contribute to poor health, and the approach to disease prevention and health promotion must include action at those levels. Dr. Quinn has served as an answer to many of those challenges by abundantly providing his time, talent, and expertise. His passion to improve health outcomes in Mississippi has positioned him to be a valuable partner in promoting the health of all Mississippians, but especially for underrepresented minority populations. It has been my pleasure to partner with Dr. Quinn to protect and promote the health of our community.

Victor D. Sutton, PhD, MPPA. Director, Ofc of Preventive Health, MS State Dept. of Health

Dr. Quinn is a true advocate for a healthier Mississippi. His dedication and commitment to Mississippians, especially those who are stricken by poverty, has not gone unnoticed by many in the Mississippi Legislature. Many thanks for his efforts to make Mississippi a healthier state!

Representative Sonya Williams Barnes, District 119, Chair, MS Legislative Black Caucus

Dr. Timothy Quinn is an influential and irreplaceable part of Mississippi's health-care system. As chairperson of my health-care task force, he has worked hard to increase health awareness and affect countless lives throughout the great City of Jackson. Dr. Quinn's excellence is showcased in his discipline to the craft of medicine and his dedication to service.

Mayor Tony T. Yarber, Jackson, MS

When we talk about the medicine, we need to address Mississippi's epidemics of bad health and health disparities. The answer is leadership, not pharmaceuticals. What an encouragement he is to all of us, doctors and patients alike, with his innovative, compassionate, energetic, and evidenced-based approach to all things healthy. Hooray for a better Mississippi and hooray for Dr. Quinn, who is leading the way! **Richard D. DeShazo, MD, MACP, Billy S. Guyton Distinguished Professor, Professor of Medicine and Pediatrics, The University of MS Medical Center**

Dr. Quinn is driven by a love for community, and his tenacity of spirit is evident in all he does to promote health and wellness to citizens across the metro area. Not only is he a celebrated family physician with a very successful practice but he's also quickly becoming one of Jackson's most influential community leaders. Above all, Dr. Quinn is a man on a mission to help us all be a little bit better and a little healthier. **Christopher Mims, *Senior Director, Communications and Marketing,* American Heart Association, Greater Southeast Affiliate**

I am Dr. Charles Miller, pastor of New Birth Fellowship Church located in Ridgeland, Mississippi. Dr. Timothy Quinn has a passion for helping people. His dedication toward serving the people is genuine. I am forever grateful for having a doctor such as Dr. Quinn who is not only kind and compassionate but willing to go above and beyond to ensure that his patients are satisfied. His commitment is indescribable. Thanks for all you do, Dr. Quinn! **Pastor Charles Miller, New Birth Fellowship Church**

While cardiovascular-disease mortality is declining, it remains our nation's leading cause of death, and Mississippians are dying of coronary heart disease and stroke at even greater rates than the nation. Meanwhile, incidence of obesity and diabetes is on the rise (American Heart Association, 2009b). Seventy percent of diabetics die of heart or blood-vessel disease, diabetes is currently the sixth leading cause of death in America, and obesity is deeply intertwined with both cardiovascular disease and diabetes. The prevalence of high blood pressure in African Americans is the highest in the world (AHA, Mayo Clinic Health Manager). Jackson is the capital city of Mississippi, with approximately 85 percent of its population being African Americans.

Mayor Tony T. Yarber recognized health disparities among the population of his city despite being home of three major hospitals, multiple health clinics, and a wealth of physicians. With a vision to make all of Jackson better, the Medical Task Force for a Healthier Jackson was created and appointed to Timothy Quinn, MD.

Dr. Timothy Quinn practices family medicine and is the medical director and owner of Quinn Healthcare PLLC located in metro Jackson. With over ten years in private practice, Dr. Quinn is a community leader and public figure whose primary focus and emphasis is on educating his patients and the public to create healthy lifestyles. His vision and leadership is helping Mississippians learn how to begin healthy living by maintaining a healthy diet and developing a regular physical-fitness routine—resulting in overall mind, body, and soul wellness.

Dr. Quinn has lectured extensively on the topics of physical fitness and obesity prevention. Since 2010, Quinn Healthcare has serviced over 22,506 patients and believes health and wellness are the true keys to a successful life. He desires to empower the community through education and physical fitness to combat obesity and its link to many illnesses.

As the chairperson of Mayor Tony T. Yarber's Task Force for a Healthier Jackson, Dr. Quinn engaged the community and orchestrated successful screenings that led to referrals to see a physician. Engaging local congregations, the task force was able to offer free screening to more than two thousand individuals. He also led two major community events for entire families where more than a thousand people were given the opportunity to take advantage of free dental, vision, and other health screenings. He accomplished this by working with the University of Mississippi Medical Center, local nursing schools, and other community stakeholders. While the community benefitted greatly, the student workers were afforded exposure and experience in the field of medicine, providing patrons, at many instances, lifesaving information. In addition to the community work, Dr. Quinn provides oversight to the City of Jackson employee clinic set in place by the Yarber administration. This clinic provides medical services to city employees and their family members free of charge. Prior to the implementation of this clinic, Dr. Quinn and the task force provided medical screening for city employees, and the results assisted in shaping the narrative as to why the implementation of this free employee health clinic was necessary.

Elis L. McBride, **Special Projects Coordinator, City of Jackson**